Brain Fog

A Practical Guide to Banishing Brain Fog

(Everything Entrepreneurs Need to Know About Overcoming Brain Fog)

Donald Valenzuela

Published By **Tyson Maxwell**

Donald Valenzuela

All Rights Reserved

Brain Fog: A Practical Guide to Banishing Brain Fog (Everything Entrepreneurs Need to Know About Overcoming Brain Fog)

ISBN 978-1-7752436-0-1

No part of this guidebook shall be reproduced in any form without permission in writing from the publisher except in the case of brief quotations embodied in critical articles or reviews.

Legal & Disclaimer

The information contained in this book is not designed to replace or take the place of any form of medicine or professional medical advice. The information in this book has been provided for educational & entertainment purposes only.

The information contained in this book has been compiled from sources deemed reliable, and it is accurate to the best of the Author's knowledge; however, the Author cannot guarantee its accuracy and validity and cannot be held liable for any errors or omissions. Changes are periodically made to this book. You must consult your doctor or get professional medical advice before using any of the suggested remedies, techniques, or information in this book.

Upon using the information contained in this book, you agree to hold harmless the Author from and against any damages, costs, and expenses, including any legal fees potentially resulting from the application of any of the information provided by this guide. This disclaimer applies to any damages or injury caused by the use and application, whether directly or indirectly, of any advice or information presented, whether for breach of contract, tort, negligence, personal injury, criminal intent, or under any other cause of action.

You agree to accept all risks of using the information presented inside this book. You need to consult a professional medical practitioner in order to ensure you are both able and healthy enough to participate in this program.

Table Of Contents

Chapter 1: What is Stress? 1

Chapter 2: What is Brain Fog? 15

Chapter 3: What are the negative health risks that could be a result from stress that are prolonged? 21

Chapter 4: How do we understand the main consequences of stress on the brain? 29

Chapter 5: How do you manage stress? for managing stress? 39

Chapter 6: 5 weeks for dealing with stress and beat Brain Fog 69

Chapter 7: The Importance of Optimum Mental Health in Today's World 87

Chapter 8: Causes of Brain Fog 96

Chapter 9: How Brain Fog Affects Your Personal and Professional Life 103

Chapter 10: The Work Environment 112

Chapter 11: Learn to Think Straight 121

Chapter 12: Brain Power Food 127

Chapter 13: Physical Exercise 176

Chapter 1: What is Stress?

There's no definitive definition of stress, as it is a subject that differs according to perception of the concept. But, the most widely used and accepted definition of stress can be said to mean that "stress is a mental phenomenon that results from pressure." Certain psychologists consider stress to be a relation between a person with the surroundings that is evaluated as the person who exceeds the limits of his or her capabilities and placing their health in peril.

If we're upset by things, a variety of physiological and emotional reactions occur. A few of the triggers that lead to stress are the loss of a family member as well as illness, loss of a spouse or partner, loss of employment and many other.

But, keep in mind that certain circumstances may not necessarily be stress-inducing for another person therefore, the signs of stress may not can be applied to everybody. There is a myriad of demands and pressures that cause stress on a person's daily life. They are also regarded as symptoms of stress. The stressors are not just because of negative events however, they can also be related to events that are positive. Stress on one's ability to adjust and deal to new circumstances can be an indication of stress.

Things to Know:

They aren't always caused by external factors. Self-esteem issues and unrealistic or unrealistic goals, perfectionists, extreme or suppressed anger, and constant critique are just a few symptoms of stress. They all fall in the category of stressors that are internal. But, there are typical external stressors that can be seen as good indicators of stress.

Significant changes to an individual's life may be a significant source of anxiety. A few of the most important shifts include moving to a new location or a child moving abroad for school, pregnancy or a diagnosis of a life-threatening illness like cancer and AIDS. Each of these situations are typical symptoms of stress within the life of an individual.

Furthermore to this, there are many factors that cause stress as a result of life every day, such as the surroundings that a person lives in as well as relationships with friends and relatives, stress at work as well as societal stress.

There are a variety of signs that indicate stress. But, the three most prominent indicators of stress are an person who is easily angry as well as a failure to focus and keep a concentration on the issue instead of the daily activities.

Other indicators of stress include stress, fatigue, sleep issues and irritation. They can also be a sign of addiction to substances or alcohol, excessive eating, or eating nothing in any way mood swings, and other symptoms. In the end, it's essential to keep in mind that at the beginning, people should not overlook the indicators of stress to avoid the possibility of future issues.

A few statistics on Stress

Stress is an all-encompassing issue across all of the United States and around the globe. Within the U.S., a 2012 study conducted in collaboration with the American Psychological Association revealed important findings and effects on brain function as well as general well-being. In the "Stress in America" study 220 people aged between 18 and 67 years old or more were asked to take part in the survey. The following findings are especially concerning:

The way we live and our behavior is responsible for many of the challenges for the stretched health system.

19 percent of Americans consider their healthcare as being of high health care of good quality.

Just 22% of people say their healthcare provider aids the management of anxiety.

A third of patients who suffer from high stress do not discuss their managing their stress with their doctor while 73% agreed the management of their stress was essential.

Over the past 5 years, 60 percent of people have attempted to manage stress, but just 47% are convinced that they've been successful.

The study uncovered the most significant sources of stress, including:

There isn't enough funds (69 percent)

Problems with work (65 percent)

The economy (61 percent)

Obligations of the family (57 percent)

Relations (56 percent)

Health problems in the family (52 percent)

Health concerns for individuals (51 percent)

Which of the following affect you the most? Each of these, but with a few exceptions, including the economy, have something to do with be related to the way you conduct yourself. If you take the right method and the right effort, all could be modified significantly, and can all be altered at least in some manner. The trend is troubling, with a rise in women experiencing anxiety. A majority of women (43%) are experiencing increased stress during the past 5 years, while 33% of males.

Do you see a link between stress and chronic illnesses? Of the 220 people surveyed 70 percent were diagnosed with at least one of the following ailments such as heart disease or attack or heart attack, high blood pressure Type 1 diabetes or Type 2 diabetes high cholesterol, cancer excess weight or obesity as well as asthma, stroke or other respiratory diseases or disorders of anxiety, depression or chronic pain or arthritis.

Despite more frequent visits with their physician, for patients who suffer from these chronic ailments, only 25% said the health professional was extremely helpful helping them manage the stress.

Are you aware that chronic illness could influence brain function? Do you think you could be experiencing Brain Fog can be caused due to these conditions? Are there any things you can take to reduce the fog in your brain, enhance the health of your brain and slow the progression or onset of chronic illnesses? Find out more here.

Recent research suggests an average of 43% the adults living in the United States suffer from adverse consequences from physical stress. Additionally, between 75% and 90 percent of doctor consults involve health issues that are a result of stress. Also, it was found that stress-related physical symptoms are associated with six major causes of death including suicide, lung problems and cirrhosis of the liver and cancer, as well as accidents and heart disease, etc.

Though stress may have negative consequences for the body, all forms of stress can be beneficial. Imagine how our lives would be like if we didn't feel any pressure? In the absence of stress, the way we go about carrying out activities will be identical and no effort is put into one task in comparison to the other. There are two main types of stress, good tension and negative stress.

Good Stress and Bad Stress

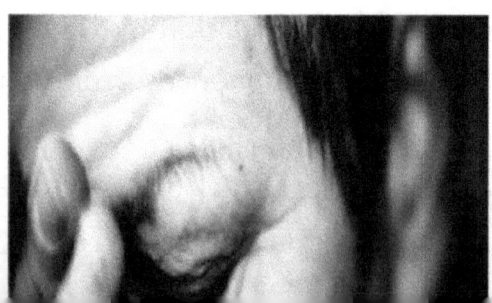

The feeling of stress is normal since our brains register this information and sends out the appropriate chemical signals that give us the needed boost in dealing any stressful or stress circumstance. A variety of experts on stress concur that small to moderate levels of stress increase the senses and help to fight off infection in order for us to be able to carry out tasks with efficiency. Psychologists refer to these as 'good stressful events'. If there is no good stress, the human body does not have the capacity to cope with the necessary fight or fight response that is essential for coping with various difficult or dangerous situations.

If you're cognizant of the fact that even a little or moderate stress can be harmful to humans There is a different form of stress, called 'bad stress'. Stress is considered to be bad when humans experience stress in high amounts or over a long duration of time, such as over a period of several weeks, or over a period of time, like for months.

The stress that is caused by this type of situation is linked with a range of ailments, including depression, high blood pressure and asthma, heart diseases as well as other. Also that the quantity and long-term stress which puts a person in physical and emotional danger is known as high stress.

The Effects of Stress on Health

Based on the U.S. Department of Health and Human Services National Institute of Health There are three primary kinds of stress that can cause the risk of mental and physical health:

* The stress of the day that is associated with pressures from family working, and the other obligations

* The anxiety that can come when a drastic change occurs like the loss of a job, divorce, or illness the loss of the job

* Traumatic stress occurs most often when an event occurs such as attack, war, accident, or natural disaster where a person their loved ones are injured or in danger of dying.

Human bodies respond to this type of stress in the same way, However, individuals may experience tension in a different way. In particular, certain sufferers may have digestive issues but others could experience extreme symptoms of insomnia, headaches, or sleeplessness as well as anger, depression and insanity. Though the impact of stress on the body vary depending on the individual however, here are some frequent effects of stress for the human body.

• Lower back lower back pain

* Chest pain

* Sweaty palms

* Increased heart rate beat

* Indigestion problems

* Excessive sweating

* Diarrhea

* Bad breath

* Sick stomach

* Retinopathy in the neck or shoulders

* Stomach or abdominal pain

* Muscle spasms

* Skin irritations and unidentified skin rashes

A variety of easily identifiable signs can be a sign that someone experiencing high amounts of stress. If you are experiencing one of the signs listed below, you must immediately take steps to lessen the anxiety-producing factors before they become dangerous.

Here are some common signs of stress:

* Obesity, over-eating and obesity

* Excessive consumption or increase in the amount of alcohol

* Unability to focus

* Anger that is suppressed or increased

• Inability to take simple choices

* A lack of Humor

* Paranoia

* Unstable work

• Loss of control over the emotions

• Lack of curiosity

• Loss of appetite

* More smoking

• Increased consumption of coffee

* Excessive irritability

* Insomnia or excessive sleeping

* Feeling of apathy

* Nail Biting

Stress from physical causes not just affects the body of a person and brain, but it affects them also. The brain isn't functioning well when we're overwhelmed. This causes a condition called brain fog', also known as cognitive dysfunction that impacts thousands of people at any given time. In the following chapter we'll analyze this problem more in depth and examine what it does to the human body, and how it affects the daily day life of a particular.

Chapter 2: What is Brain Fog?

Brain fog, also known as cognitive dysfunction, can be described as an affliction of the mind that causes mental confusion or a lack of clarity that could be due to ongoing or extended stress or a underlying health condition. When we experience an uneasy brain due to fog that is caused by constant tension and stress that we are unable to perform efficiently in our day-to everyday tasks. It is often associated with an lack of focus or recall small information.

What causes this? In simple terms, concentration levels may be diminished enough that machines or driving a vehicle could be dangerous. Brain fog sufferers can easily become distracted. Each day tasks are more challenging. It can become very embarrassing and stressful. One could be looking for their wallet only to find it hidden in the freezer. What caused that? It was a case of brain fog.

How prevalent is Brain Fog?

The brain fog that plagues many people, which includes infants as well as adults. This can cause daily issues and unhappiness in relationships. It may cause extreme frustration as well as a lack of ability to perform in a social setting.

The Four Major Causes of Brain Fog

* Stress: It is the most common factor that causes the fog in your brain. Stress overstimulates the brain and causes damage to nerve cells which causes brain fog.

* Fatigue: It is another main cause for headaches. The effects of fatigue also impact the gray matter inside the brain, which can lead to various mental diseases.

* Nutrient Deficiencies: Another important causes of the fog in your brain are nutritional deficiencies. The brain needs all essential nutrients for proper functioning. But a diet lacking in vital nutrients, such as

magnesium, vitamin B-12 and amino acids can hinder normal brain function and robs your brain of oxygen creating brain fog.

* Depression: Many people around the world are suffering from depression. The disorder causes problems in concentration and making the right decisions. These can be attributed to the signs from brain fog.

The Common Symptoms of Brain Fog

Because of the inscrutable character of brain fog, or cognitive impairment It can be difficult to spot the signs. Someone who suffers from cognitive impairment often is aware that they're unwell and that their brain appears confused. The following are the more common signs experienced by those experiencing brain fog.

A lack of mental clarity

* Impossibility to concentrate or concentrate

* Feelings of mental fuzzyness

* A decrease in focus

• Trouble remembering details of the names, dates, and events and other details

* Mental fatigue

While these are the most common signs of brain fog, it's essential to remember that the symptoms can vary from one person to another individual. In addition to the signs mentioned in the above list, someone who is suffering from brain fog might have feelings of depression as well.

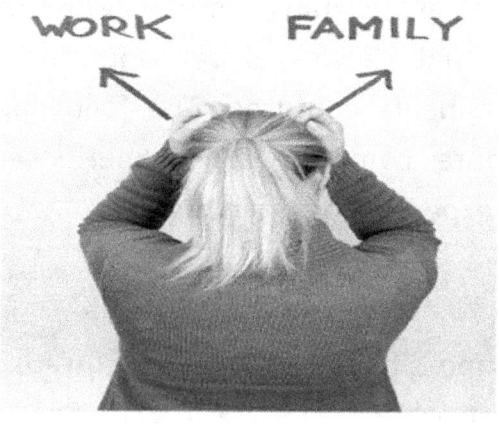

The Effects of Brain Fog on Human Beings

Relationship problems There is an overwhelmingly YES. It is well-known that brain fog can be a factor in lower self-esteem. Low self-esteem can cause numerous relationship difficulties and could cause further issues, eventually destroying these relationships.

Professional issues: As we've discussed before that brain fog causes decreased ability to focus. A person with brain fog has it hard to read or retain what they read. Concentration levels for individuals are diminished enough that they find it hard to perform their job and puts their job or their job in peril. For those who want to put it into easy terms, a person could lose their job due to the fog of their brains.

The reasons for the fog in your brain are many and may be physical as well as emotional. In terms of the cause physical of the fog in the brain, long-term stress is believed as the main reason for brain fog. Stress that is prolonged does not just cause brain fog however, it also causes adverse consequences on body organs as well as the general health and wellbeing of individuals. In the next section we'll explore the negative physical effects that stress can have on our health.

Chapter 3: What are the negative health risks that could be a result from stress that are prolonged?

Stress that is prolonged can have a significant adverse effect on your health. Most people believe that stress is an emotional condition, but few people realize that stress can cause illness and injuries. It can also cause serious harm to all the organs and systems of the body. In this article, we will explore the effects of stress over time on the essential organs of our body.

The effects on our bodies - The lungs, the arteries, the heart and liver (alcohol medication)

What effects does stress have on the heart?

Stress stimulates the automatic component that controls the nerve system. This affects various organs, which includes the heart. The prolonged stress can increase the rate of pumping or activity of the heart. This elevates blood pressure and increases the likelihood of suffering from cardiovascular illnesses.

Affects of stress on arterial arteries

The arteries are triggered by stress to contract, which results in the intima-medial thickness. This is the measurement of arteries. Constrictions in arterial arteries caused by stress reduces circulation of blood towards the heart. This puts individuals at chance of suffering from heart attacks.

The effects of stress on the lungs

Lungs play a role in receiving oxygen and transferring it through the body. Stress raises the rate of the lungs taking oxygen. This is why people experience rapid breathing as oxygen flows into the body at a quicker speed, which results in the heart beating faster. Stress can increase circulation of blood into the body by up to 400 percent.

The effects of stress on the liver

Stress from emotional causes stress on the liver. Additionally, many suffering from stress use drugs to relieve anxiety. The thing that many people aren't aware of is that medication is processed by the liver. The excessive consumption of stress relief medications could harm the liver. Drinkers who consume alcohol as a way to alleviate anxiety or stress can directly affect their livers. Anyone who drinks excessively and taking stressing medications for the liver is more at danger of sustaining damage to the liver.

Stress hormones and its effects

Stress affects all the hormones that are present in the body of a person. Stress, for instance, releases cortisol, which is a key hormone that is produced from the adrenal glands that performs functions including regular glucose metabolism, the regulation of blood pressure in addition to immune function and inflammation response.

The hormonal effects of hormones - the dangers of cortisol

The Dangers of Cortisol

Obesity

Cortisol's release in people who suffer from chronic tension increases the amount of abdominal fat. It also acts as the principal link between the stressor and the weight increase. Furthermore, someone experiencing stress could experience anxiety-related cravings for food.

In particular, stress is frequently associated with the weight gain of a person because someone experiencing stress will develop a craving for salt, fats as well as sugar, to alleviate the tension. In the end, they gain weight which eventually results in overweight. The weight gain comes due to abdominal fat. It also can increase the chance of developing anxiety and heart conditions.

Memory Loss

Along with making someone overweight, cortisol from stress can also have other negative impacts on the general health of an individual. In the long run, for instance elevated cortisol levels can cause elevated blood pressure in addition to diabetes and pre-diabetes as well as causing changes to the brain which affect memory. Human studies have demonstrated that cortisol levels induced by stress affect the

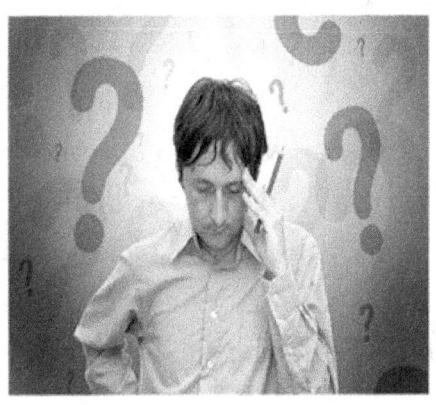

consolidation over time of the memory of declarative information.

Memory loss occurs as cortisol causes shrinkage of the brain's memory centre which is located within the hippocampus. The loss of the hippocampus to damage is also among the first symptoms of Alzheimer's disease. It is which is a form of degenerative dementia that progresses or memory loss that occurs when the person's memory is deteriorated, which is followed by impairment in thinking and speech and eventually, complete insanity.

In addition to weight gain and loss of memory Higher and longer-lasting levels of cortisol within the bloodstream of a person who is stressed out regularly can cause the negative side effects of:

* High Blood Pressure

* Cognitive impairment

* Blood sugar imbalances

* Thyroid function is suppressed.

* The increase in bad cholesterol or LDL, and decreased quantities of the good cholesterol, or HDL

* Heart attacks

* Strokes

* An increase in belly fat

* Inflammation and immune system declines. response

* Slower healing of wounds

Stress is a major factor in the health of all the vital organs in the body. But, the effects of stress are more severe in the brain. Stress overloads the brain with high-powered hormones. The cumulative impact of these hormones can damage or destroys brain cells which can lead to loss of memory. In the next section we'll analyze the effect of stress on brain cells.

Chapter 4: How do we understand the main consequences of stress on the brain?

Recent research has shown that prolonged stress has a devastating effect upon the brain. Research has shown that stress-related hormones alter mental structure of the brain to the extent that affects learning mood, and memory. Furthermore many additional effects that stress can have on the brain. Some of which are listed below:

The cognitive symptoms of stress

Human psychology states that cognition, or thinking, is a complex process that involves many steps that involve perception, consciousness, associations, and memory. Stress affects the performance of different areas of the brain, which are responsible for the cognitive activities as well as alters the performance of areas of the brain that are involved in emotional states. Stress also interferes with cognitive functions of the brain on various levels. It can cause diverse cognitive signs like insomnia as well as racing thoughts, mental blurring, difficulties in making decisions or preoccupation, and memory difficulties. Here are a few of the main cognitive symptoms that stress can cause.

Memory issues

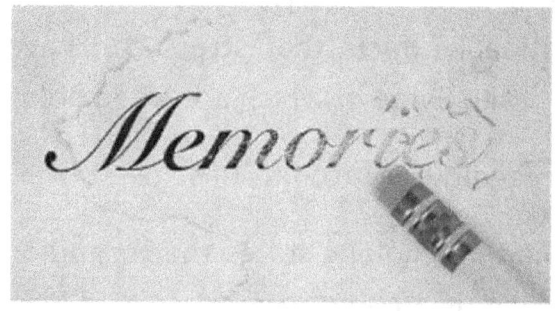

The connection between stress and memory loss or loss is widely known. Research suggests that high levels of cortisol released during stressful circumstances can damage the neural connections that connect brain cells. In the preceding chapter, increased levels of cortisol hormone that causes stress disrupts memory. Stressors can cause lapses in concentration. In the end, the person will not be able to retain information as the brain is not able to focus on the topic initially. Additionally stress damages or kills the cells of diverse brain areas.

Disabilities to focus

Stress and concentration for long periods don't go together. The relationship between concentration and stress is in inverse proportional. When a person is spending more being stressed and pressure, their capacity to focus diminishes. Stress triggers the release of another hormone associated with stress, adrenaline. The adrenaline hormone boosts the sensitivity of our brain until it becomes aware of everything that happens within a specific individual. The result is that a person can become frequently lost in their surroundings. What's wrong with this lies in the way that brain struggles against itself whenever the person is trying to focus or is trying to get their things done. This affects the capability of a person to complete their work and, in turn, affects the level of concentration in individuals.

Poor judgment

Stress may lead to poor judgment. It prevents people from taking the right decisions, and can cause people to ignore their own interests and wants. Stress, as we've seen earlier, causes individuals to be focused. It is made worse by stress-related headaches. A lack of concentration and poor judgement can lead to difficulties at work. Stress-related poor judgment can affect the capacity of an individual to make logical decisions. A person is unable to make the right decision. This is why the person makes bad choices in the workplace and at home. This can have a detrimental effects on their personal life as well and professional life.

The pessimistic outlook or the thoughts

Other signs of stress in the brain are negative or pessimistic thinking. When stressed, a person engages in self-talk that is irrational, not able to believe in perfection and is unable to accept the abilities of everyone. This self-talk may lead to emotional turmoil and an naive mind that causes the individual to miss possibilities in life, and avoid solutions to issues in the world in general and act against what goals one would like to achieve in their life.

The thoughts of anxiety or racing thoughts

Racing thoughts are a result of stress in particular in the evening. Though some individuals may mistake regular thoughts with race thoughts Racing thoughts are ones that are hard to manage and prevent people from sleeping. They cause anxiety, and hinder the ability of an individual to concentrate as well as cause anxiety and shame. While racing thoughts may be not a cause for concern, it's how a person reacts who is affected by them that could cause more danger. If the circumstances are extreme one may experience be in a state of panic, and it can be difficult to keep their thoughts under control. These things can create a huge amount of anxiety.

Continuously worried

Another significant cognitive manifestation of stress is the constant worry. Worrying refers to the feeling of unease or being too worried over a particular issue or circumstance. In the event of stress, both the body and mind of the person go into hyperdrive, and they are constantly focused on "what might happen." Worse than constant worrying is that one worries about fears that are not real and this only increases worry. Someone who is constantly in anxiety is usually extremely sensitive to their surroundings and perceives nearly everything, everyone or anything in the vicinity as a danger. The negative impact of worry is substantial in that it affects the everyday life of an person and can affect sleep patterns as well as relationships, daily routines eating habits, and work performance.

The Effects of Stress on Areas of the Brain

Here are the most frequent cognitive signs that are caused by stress. They are typically caused by stress can affect the different areas within the brain. Long-term exposure to stress can have detrimental effects on every major part in the brain.

* Effect of Stress on the Hippocampus

The hippocampus is component of the limbic system. The limbic system comprises an array of brain structures that are located around the stem of brain. The hippocampus is of neurons, with a variety of branches that resemble dendrites and axons. They form connections with different brain neurons. The brain's limbic system generally and the hippocampus particular are crucial when dealing with emotions like fear, anger as well as motivations and memories. The

Hippocampus is also used to store, retrieve and stores new memories. It's also the only area of brain that is known to generate new neurons which is a process called neurogenesis. Stressors like cortisol adversely affects the hippocampus through reducing its dimensions. A shrinkage or injury to the hippocampus due to stress hormones alters an individual's ability to retain and remember data, leading to loss of memory. In the extreme, stress hormones may also boost the number of cells dying within the hippocampus.

Recent studies have shown that long-term exposure to cortisol can hinder the ability of the hippocampus undergo neurogenesis. Additionally, since the hippocampus and other limbic structures within the brain also play a role to overcome fear-related responses that are triggered by chronic stress can also find it hard to conquer their anxiety.

The effect of stress on dendrites

Dendrites are small branch-like structures found in neurons of the brain. Their main purpose dendrites is sending signals and also receive them. Research suggests that stress causes hormones to shrink dendrites. This means that what information dendrites receive are not transmitted through nerve cells. The result is a high level of anxiety for the individual. A study was that was conducted in 2011 it was determined that loss of dendrites is one major reasons for increased anxiety levels.

Stress can have an effect on the amygdala

The amygdala is a different part of the brain which is in the process of being affected by stress. It regulates fear as well as other emotions. The amygdala is triggered by stress to increase in size and shrink dendrites within the hippocampus. Studies have proven the two effects of stress are the main cause of increased anxiety. When stress causes the amygdala's size to grow in size, an individual is more anxious and afraid. Additionally, the amygdala grows for those suffering from chronic depression.

Stress can have an effect on Prefrontal Cortex

The prefrontal cortex of the brain is a part which is responsible for the emotion as well as self-control, and also physiological function. The prefrontal cortex supports the most advanced cognitive capabilities and is also the region of the brain which is most susceptible to the negative consequences of stress. There is evidence that suggests even the smallest amount of acute, inexplicably unbearable stress triggers alteration in the dendrites of the prefrontal. In one study, it was observed that stress can result in cognitive, biochemical and morphological modifications to the cortex of prefrontal. Additionally, changes caused by stress impact the functioning that the brain's prefrontal cortex performs, and can cause impairment in working memory.

Chapter 5: How do you manage stress? for managing stress?

It's hard for anyone to lead a regular life in the absence of knowing how to manage anxiety, particularly when there are new challenges to face daily. That is the cause of an increasing rate of heart attacks and strokes among young people as they face a variety of problems at once.

A lot of people aren't just ignorant of strategies to deal the stress issue, but they're unaware that stress can be the cause of depression, obesity hair loss, and sleep deprivation. The majority of people are worried about the mounting cost of their bills as well as rising fuel costs and other issues that affect their lives that cause them to be stressed.

Strategies to Manage Stress:

It is essential to know what triggers stress and strategies to manage stress. It is equally essential to pinpoint the main source of stress since it will allow a person create strategies to cope the stress. One of the most crucial things to be aware of is that you can't always eliminate the stressors. In the case of a anxiety is caused by a bill which was the result of an emergency, and the invoice is not paid, it could be sent to collections, causing more hassles. The bill could only be an incredibly small cost to your pocket, but should you settle the bill on time and on time, you'll be relieved from stressing over the issue.

When your situation gets way out of control If things get out of hand, it is possible immediately seek assistance from a medical expert. You might be suffering from stress that is excessive when it is not addressed this can result in grave health problems; if not treated, anxiety-related problems could result in substance use disorder or suicidal thoughts, which are common symptoms of stress for students in these times.

You will find a variety of solutions to manage stress. In particular, figuring out how to prioritize tasks and set schedules can help manage stress in a significant way. There are many exercises like exercising, swimming and video games, joining a club, among other rejuvenating methods to reduce anxiety.

The other important methods to deal stress include eating a healthy diet and getting enough rest both of which allow you to manage stress better and more effectively.

If you're experiencing extreme amounts of stress, do not be afraid to take courses on how to manage anxiety without a second thought. Once you've mastered these techniques and techniques, you'll have more control of your feelings.

Positive and positive thoughts that can ease the stress of your life significantly. It is essential to examine the elements that cause stress, and take the appropriate actions to reduce and manage your stress levels. A variety of stress management programs are accessible via adult education classes at high schools in the area or at community colleges.

Techniques for managing stress effectively aid in reducing the adverse effects of stress as well as provide better control over depression. Strategies for managing stress do not just aid in dealing with stress-inducing moments in life however, they also assist in create a positive outlook. Strategies for stress management establish guidelines and set standards that aid people manage and calm the stress. Strategies for stress management also help you to achieve your objectives.

Find help from a licensed medical professional who specializes in mental health

It is essential to speak with a licensed health practitioner in the event of a need for medications. The doctor may recommend an benzodiazepine, a stress-reducing medication that are in the category of anti-anxiety. It is usually prescribed by doctors in a brief time frame to decrease or stop anxiety.

A doctor may recommend diazepam. However, it is only prescribed in cases where the patient is affected by stress. The doctor may prescribe different forms of medication for stress, like antidepressants or antipsychotics in accordance with the severity of stress. But, it is important to be aware of the possible side consequences of these drugs such as dizziness and rapid breathing, an increased blood pressure, sweating too much or body aches, as well as an increase in the feelings of despair, panic and anxiety. Because of this, it's not advised to use medications as your first treatment for anxiety or stress.

In general, the side effects associated with medication for stress can be managed when you keep in touch your doctor. Your physician is the only person who can determine which type of medication which is most suitable for your needs. It is essential to disclose your daily routine and medical history as this data could make a difference to your treatment of stress. When you get the proper guidance on these drugs from your psychiatrist and you'll be free of stress and lead the life you want to live in a healthy and regular way.

Peer Support

Studies have proven that talking with someone regarding your stress or problems can greatly ease this anxiety. Therefore, if you are feeling anxious, you should talk to someone you trust; keep close to those who are able to provide emotional and additional support. Support from your relatives, friends and communities or religious groups will yield amazing results.

If you are uncomfortable sharing their concerns with others can keep a diary where they write in their journals all the issues they face as well as stress-producing factors. It is important to remember that writing in itself is an exercise that can assist you in relieving anxiety.

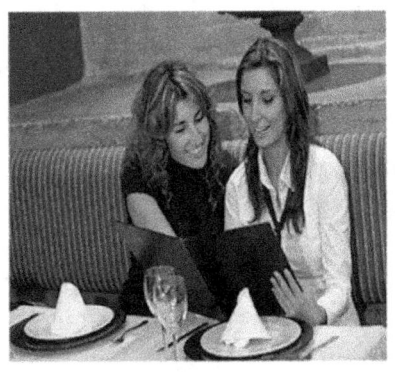

A number of people have been able overcome their anxiety by using counselors who are professionals and peer-to-peer support. Take a real instance from our lives:

Over the years, Mary Jones, a single mother of a two year old son as well as working at a new place of work had difficulty to stay focused on her job. It was disrupting her sleep, and for the majority times, she was overwhelmed.

Mary discovered that she had not been connecting with her fellow students and she was socially unengaged and felt very lonely. In the wake of this realization she immediately contacted her closest friend she was delighted to talk with Mary after an extended period of time. Following their conversation, Mary also decided to get professional help. It was a huge success. Mary managed to create the routine she had established and alter her outlook after speaking to a therapist.

Laughter

In the case of managing stress, there's not any better way to do it than with laughter. A few more giggles is all is needed to ease the stress. One of the main benefits of laughter therapy lies in the fact it slows down the stress response, and boosts blood circulation, thereby which gives you a relaxing feeling.

It also assists in reducing muscle tension and reduces physical signs of stress. Thoughts that are negative, arising due to chemical reactions that take place in our bodies as a result of stress will only cause more stress. Conversely, laughter produces neuropeptides. They fight stress and enable you to manage stressful or difficult circumstances by allowing you to be in touch with others.

Here's how therapy with laughter can help Alex get through anxiety:

Alex seldom left his workstation in his workplace, and was often having lunch as well as dinner at the same time. A few days ago, Alex received a call from his wife who told his wife that he'd forgotten to turn the burner of gas on the cooker on while he was leaving to work. It wasn't the first occasion that Alex was unable to remember something; just recently it was when he forgot to shut the door to the refrigerator unlocked all through the night. Alex began to notice that he had lost concentration and becoming less attentive. To his advantage, Alex's workplace had arranged one of its own Employee Assistance Program (EAP). With the programme, Alex came to know how stress affects the memory of an individual. When he learned about the harmful consequences of stress Alex made the decision to not work whenever it was not urgent, and opted to spend time with his colleagues in the office, and with his wife at minimum once a week. Alex enjoyed comedy, so his wife and he took a movie to watch and went to catch comedy performances at the local comedy club. After a period of four weeks, following the pattern, Alex realized that his recall had decreased.

Exercise

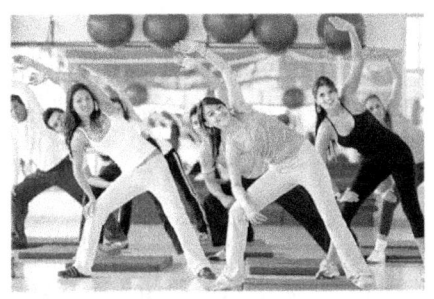

In accordance with numerous research studies, exercising helps people to live healthier. It makes your body and mind fresher, and leads to better sleeping. A lot of people worry about their appearance. However, regardless of whether this is an issue, being physically active will help ease anxiety. Stress can affect the physical as well as mental wellbeing.

An extended jogging routine with a vigorous yoga session or refreshing water after working a long day is a great way to reduce stress and live the life of peace.

Everyday activities could result in stress, and even ailments like heart diseases as well as diabetes, among others. Training is the ideal way to reduce stress. Here are a few of the routines you could perform every day to help keep from stress

* Yoga: Yoga improves flexibility, builds muscles and, perhaps most important it eases breathing and decreases anxiety. A few basic breathing exercises will help you relax and reduce anxiety.

Breathing exercises and meditation breathing exercises bring many advantages. One of the best things about breathing exercises is that you can practice them at any time and at any time you're feeling overwhelmed. All you have to do is breathe normally and with a slightly more intense exhale. Also, you can regularly engage in meditation exercises that require deep breathing, such as meditation for the advantages that they bring in letting go of tension.

Regular meditation sessions help maintain the body and mind of a person unaffected by stress. Stress meditation is proven to be among the best methods to treat those who suffer from stress. Additionally, meditation can help maintain the proper balance of psychological and emotional state of our minds.

The meaning of meditation is different depending on the context in which its application. The practice began as a religion-based practice. Hinduism is believed to be the primary source of its origin. Since the beginning, many were using meditation to relieve stress during yoga.

The Simple Way to Meditate

As you meditate it is important to maintain a good posture. Thus, it is important to take a seat in a comfortable position and close your eyes. Focus upon a specific image or sound, and relax with deep breaths. Repeat this practice for at minimum 20 minutes each day. The majority of stress relieving products have a variety of adverse effects.

Stress meditation is not a risk in any way, because it's a natural and effective method of healing to manage anxiety.

Finding Meditation Classes

There is a possibility that you can locate mediation classes in the local high school, community college, or university.

If you're struggling to locate suitable classes for meditation or you don't have time for meditation then you could take a listen to the audio files available:

Techniques for relaxation - Total relaxation is the most effective method to exercise the entire body, particularly in times when you feel like you have a lot of stress. Relaxation techniques relax your mind and body. The only thing you need to do is to stop any task you're doing then relax, and take a slow breathing. If you are able to afford it then you could also opt for an expert massage. Massage is also regarded for its relaxing effects and helps to reduce anxiety.

How Cathy got rid of brain fog through exercises and relaxation techniques

In the morning, Cathy opened her eyes after a brief nap. She had slept poorly throughout the previous months. It was affecting her ability to concentrate and remember.

When she was employed at an accounting company, she worked with math and figures on a regular day basis. However, over the last couple of days, Cathy noticed that her capacity to deal with figures had diminished.

The woman was unable to figure out basic statistics. It was actually the brain fog that caused the insomnia. In her 28th year She realized there was no way to diagnose dementia. stress was the cause. negatively impacting her life, both personal professional lives. Cathy took the decision to address her sleep disorder. She joined the five-week relaxation program and made a decision to not engage in activities like viewing TV prior to getting ready to go to bed. Within two weeks Cathy could be more focused and realize that the fog in her brain was totally removed.

Therapy for floatation

Floatation therapy is extensively used to treat stress. It has been proven in research that suggests the reduction of the stress and pain with floatation therapy. Floatation therapy is primarily about drifting in an environment that is gravity-free. The practice relieves anxiety and pain by eliminating all pressure and gravity off your body. It not only relieves physical discomfort, but also stimulates your mental thinking. It allows you to completely unwind and relax, while your concentration and creative thinking are stimulated.

The research shows that just an hour of flotation has an effect comparable to 4 hours of sleep. It is due to the fact that when we flot, our body's brain produces more slow-moving patterns. The brainwaves that are produced are called theta waves. They're most often experienced during meditation, or when you're to sleep. They are also followed by clear thought as well as the release of endorphins that are our body's natural opioids. Studies have shown that floating can help in reducing blood pressure as well as heart rate, and can be beneficial in decreasing the level of stress-related chemical levels within the body.

Writing as Therapy

Writing is another crucial aspect in controlling stress. Utilizing thought log pages or diaries for activities helps you clear any negative thoughts from your mind. The primary reason to use writing for therapy is the fact that simply writing your thoughts down on paper can provide instant relief of stress.

If you're unable to go to bed in the night, write down all concerns that pop into your thoughts. It will help you tackle those concerns at the beginning of your day. A notepad that you carry in your purse or in your pocket will mean that you are able to write whatever you want, whenever and go through what you are worried about the most. Then, you can find the solution to get rid of anxiety or for the most part, tension.

If you are considering writing as therapy to relieve anxiety, these are a few aspects you must take into consideration.

• Write about the items that make your mood in times of stress.

• Remember the things that been helpful to you when you were in the same situation.

Note down the things about that you require assistance (e.g. speak to someone or be around other people).

Note down the things you are not to do, things are based on experience and do make no sense.

Write down what you consider are your own strengths as well as resources.

Be kind and caring. Be supportive in your understanding, encouraging, and compassionate towards your own vulnerable self.

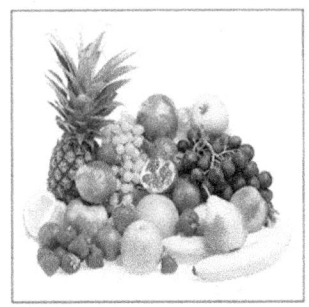

Healthful eating habits and good nutrition

Diets are often at risk in times of stress and depressed. We can also feel anxious, stressed, or overloaded by obligations. Stress can cause people to indulge in a diet of excess. In addition, when stress brings the prospect of depression and fatigue unhealthy eating can take an outstretched hand to meals which are calming or fast and

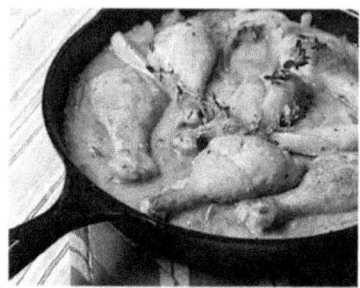

often filled with sugar and fat.

The high-calorie food items stimulate the release of chemicals within the brain which makes us feel better however only for a moment. Over time, these meals can cause psychological stress, leading into overeating, and ultimately the weight gain.

Maintaining a balanced and healthy lifestyle that is based on good nutrition an established method of keeping tension at bay in the initial in the first. But, if you're overwhelmed, here are a few steps you can do to control stress by adjusting your diet.

Get balanced food: To reduce stress, make sure you incorporate lean proteins like egg whites, or chicken within your daily food plan. Additionally, you can add food items such as meat, fish and soy-based products into your food plan. Protein fills you up and keeps you alert and focused. The perfect way to end your meals with fresh fruit as well as whole grain and vegetable.

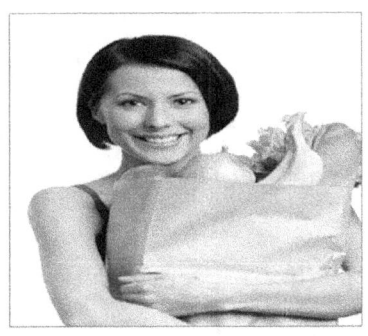

Don't skip meals If you don't have the desire to eat because tension has diminished your appetite. You may have decided to skip meals completely. If you do not consume enough food regularly, your energy levels are likely to decrease and you'll be eating excessively when you do take a break. To prevent this from happening to avoid this, don't to eat a meal in a hurry, instead, eat smaller meals regularly or regularly eat smaller portions of food over the course of the days. Stress will not be acting as a hunger killer as well as avoiding overeating and cravings for unhealthy foods that stress can trigger.

Cut back on caffeine:

When stressed, people frequently use caffeine as they believe that it will provide them with the energy needed to return to normal. But what they don't realize is that caffeine can disrupt sleep patterns, causing increased anxiety. This is why it's crucial to look for alternatives to your drink. Switch your coffee to green tea. Green tea is said to provide numerous health benefits, and it also helps in reducing stress. Stay clear of "energy drinks" which contain large quantities of caffeine and other stimulants.

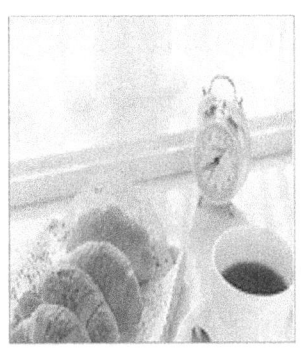

Incorporate complex carbs into your diet

Complex carbohydrates assist the brain create the chemical that makes you feel good, serotonin. The release of serotonin by the brain helps to combat anxiety. Food sources that are the most important for complex carbohydrates are:

* Whole-grain pasta

* Vegetables

* Beans

* Fruits

* Breads

* Whole-grain Cereals

* Brown Rice

* Nonfat Milk

Consume moderate quantities of healthy fats

The healthy fats in olives seeds, avocados, and avocados fatty fish aid the brain in reducing stress through the release of serotonin. We know that it's possible and straightforward to minimize the stress-related effects and to avoid the negative effects of stress through a healthy diet.

A balanced diet is a great way to combat the effects of stress through strengthening your immune system as well as lowering blood pressure. In the end it's important to adhere to an eating plan that includes the necessary nutrients and not just to lessen stress, but also to maintain the best body and mind and to live a happy lifestyle.

Supplements

An unhealthy diet, particularly an insufficient intake of specific vitamins could cause memory loss. These vitamins are reduced by drugs, illnesses alcohol or bad food regimen. If you are finding it hard to stick to a plan of eating with proper nutrition and stress relief, then you may be able to counter it by using a variety of supplements that are available. But, it's important to exercise caution and consult a doctor before taking any supplements to counter stress since there are a variety of adverse impacts. Below are some of the products that are known to combat stress.

L-Theanine

L-Theanine is an amino acids that is found primarily in leaves of green tea. These amino acids hinder the interaction of L-glutamic acid with glutamate receptors located in the brain. The characteristics of L-Theanine affect the mental state of people in stressful situations. Research has shown that the consumption of L-Theanine results in reductions in heart rate. The results of clinical studies indicate that taking L-Theanine between 50-200 mg every daily, is totally secure and acts as an anti-anxiety medication as well as a mood enhancer, which counters anxiety and other stress-related illnesses.

Casein Tryptic Hydrolysate

A new study has revealed that consumption for 30 days of tryptic hydrolsyate casein decreased anxiety-related symptoms like mental, cardiovascular and social issues and digestive issues in women.

Vitamin B12

B12 is an essential vitamin which helps to improve your memory. In addition, it's one of the main deficiency that causes memory loss. The aging process can decrease the amount of B12. A low level in Vitamin B12 can cause anemia that can cause the loss of memory.

High EPA Omega-3 Supplement

According to studies that Omega-3 fatty acids are crucial for maintaining an enlightened brain. Since our bodies do not create fatty acids Omega-3 is believed to have benefits and although it is obtainable by a healthy eating habits, it also can be taken as an effective supplement.

Ginkgo Biloba

For its role as a memory aid Ginkgo Biloba is somewhat controversial as it's believed to boost blood flow and reduce memory loss, but it can also cause adverse negative effects. Recent studies suggest that it is less effective as previously thought. More research is required.

Huperzine A

Huperzine A can improve longer-term memory, alertness in the short term as well as learning, by increasing the efficiency of neurotransmitters within the brain. This aids in the transfer of chemicals between brain cells.

Rosemary

According to the British Psychological Society's conference in the UK the researcher Dr. Mark Moss, of the University of Northumbria at Newcastle discovered that lavender and rosemary can increase memory as well as various other aspects of cognition.

Co Q-10

Co Q-10, as well as the other antioxidants like extracts of grape seeds and Vitamin E are believed to help slow down the ageing process in cells. In essence, they decrease the impact of tension on your cells. This results an overall improvement in memory.

The right diet was instrumental in helping Stacy combat the effects of stress and brain fog

At 28 Stacy believed she was in her 60s. The reason for this is that she was enduring lots of stress that was mostly due to her relationship ending and the need to accept the job that paid less. The events that were happening in her life had a negative impact on her physical health. In order to make matters worse the woman was looking to shed weight with taking stimulants. The stimulants aimed towards reducing her weight and help Stacy focus better however what was actually happening was quite the reverse. In the days, weeks, and even months Stacy could not finish her work. The rest of her sleep was a catastrophe. Actually, Stacy couldn't even remember the last time she had a restful night.

As a result of stimulants her diet was ruined and she was doing the stimulants while ignoring her food. But, her sister was aware of the problem and informed Stacy that stress was the culprit which was the cause of all the troubles in Stacy's life. Stacy discovered that she had been right and sought advice from with a nutritionist. Additionally, she started working out together with her sister. After a few months of adhering to the advice of her sister about taking vitamins such as vitamin B, working out regularly and consuming a nutritious and balanced diet, Stacy's improvement began and she saw that the brain fog that was mostly the result the stress of her life was gone.

Chapter 6: 5 weeks for dealing with stress and beat Brain Fog

After you've learned about the various elements that cause stress's toxic components It is crucial to come up with strategies to reduce your lifestyle to reduce stress. This won't just improving your general health as well as improve the quality of your brain's health as well as reduce the negative effects of brain fog.

Following the sections below in the following sections, you'll be able create a plan which is unique based on your personal experiences. It is possible to modify this plan altered as the circumstances of your life shift. Be aware that if you do not follow the make a plan, you will fall short. Therefore, it's important to give this part an amount of thought and be patient. Keep it light and fun.

When you've developed the Brain Health Action Plan, it is possible to discuss it with a different person. It could be your coworker as well as your spouse or friend or family member, as well as your physician or therapist, if you've got one. Why? Studies have shown that when you discuss your plan of action with someone else You will not just gain support in the social sphere, but also more likely to stick the plan to completion. We're ready to get going!

The 5-Week Brain Health Action Plan

Week I

The first week the goal is to identify what stressors can be affecting our lives as well as our health and the our brain. We will also seek to be cognizant of the thoughts, emotions and behaviour. There are a variety of methods that to use. The first is to keep journals to record your thoughts and feelings every daily. A different approach is to take an easy questionnaire to determine the stressors that may affect our lives. You can also ask an acquaintance or coworker about the things they observe about us, and what they think could be stressors. Whatever method you decide to use, you'll need to look for problems with regard to sleeping food and nutrition and leisure time, as well as relationship and work schedules as well as opportunities for exercise or inactivity, and methods to be able to exercise or stimulate your brain. Below are a few examples.

The Depression Anxiety Scales (DASS) is the self-reporting questionnaire with 42 questions developed to evaluate the related emotions of anxiety, depression and stress. The questionnaire is accessible to the public in the open domain. It can be reproduced here (see an appendix) to ease your way.

This is not a way to diagnose any mental health issues. Our goal is to help you identify the areas of tension and stress which you can reduce by establishing Your Brain Health Action Plan. There is also the DASS 21, which is an abbreviated form that performs very well.

People who are high-scoring on the DASS Scale

The Depression Scale

Individuals who score highly scores on the Depression Scale show the following features:

We are always optimistic regarding the future

Cannot experience pleasure

* Aren't interested in getting involved or feel uninterested

* Insistency is lacking

They are mostly convinced their lives have no meaning or significance.

* Self-disparaging

Sometimes, you feel despirited Blue, gloomy or disorientated

The Anxiety Scale

The people who have high scores On the Anxiety Scale display the following signs:

Dryness and dryness can be felt in the mouth

* Have breathing problems

* Feel the beat of your heart

Feel the palms sweating

You are always concerned about the performance of your business and a possible loss of control

Feel anxious and panicky all the time

* Tense or shaken

The Stress Scale

The people who have a high score scores on the Stress Scale show the following features:

* Can be easily affected by irritation.

* It is possible to be startled easily.

- Nervous, jittery, often fidgety

* Will not tolerate interruptions or delays

* Never over-aroused or tense.

* Restless the majority times

It is easy to become angry

Journaling

Journaling is the practice keeping a journal that allows you to explore your ideas and emotions that are a part of your daily life. Journaling can be a useful method of managing stress, provided that you write down all of your thoughts, feelings and emotions associated with stressful experiences and in full detail. This is comparable to talking about every issue with a doctor or therapy therapist, but written.

Benefits of Journaling

One of the main benefits of journaling is its ability to clear your mind and clarify your feelings. Journaling can help you discover valuable information about your own self. Additionally, it can be an excellent tool to solve problems as it helps you organize your thoughts through a thorough exploration of your emotions. Studies have shown that journaling can provide the many benefits.

* Journaling improves the cognitive function.

It can counteract some of the negative effects from stress.

* It helps strengthen the immune system and helps prevent various ailments.

Journaling can help reduce the signs of arthritis, asthma and other health issues.

Nutrition and Diet

Assessing Your Diet

A way to evaluate the quality of your food is to keep the food journal for 3 days and record everything that you eat. This can allow you to know exactly what you're eating, it can reveal the amount you're eating in reality and help you identify any issues that you're experiencing with your food. A food journal will aid you in making those necessary adjustments to aid in reducing anxiety and live a balanced and peaceful lifestyle.

Below are some helpful tips to keep track of your diet.

Note what you consume Write down every food item you consume when the food item is consumed. It includes beverages and snacks as well as water.

• List all the ingredients. Write down all the ingredients needed in the preparation of a specific food item that you consume. It is possible to list the ingredients using the format below as follows: 1/2 teaspoon salt,

1 teaspoon of honey, one tablespoon of mayonnaise, and any other ingredients that are used for the preparation of the food.

Note down the quantity/portion. It is the next step to keep track of the amount or portion of food you consume. It can be recorded using slices, ounces or tsp or other common measurement units.

Note the name of the brand When you eat cornflakes, you should include the company name, such as Kellogg's Corn Flakes or any other name. When you are drinking cold drinks make sure you list its company name, Pepsi, Coca Cola, or any other.

Be aware of what you are eating Take note of whether the food you're eating was freshly cooked or was stored in the fridge.

* The method of cooking used The method you that was used for cooking your meal. Note whether the meal that you ate was cooked in a fryer or broiled, boil baking, cooked or broiled by some other technique.

When you've recorded all of the above on your food journal for 3 days, it's time to review the journal. The diary can be analyzed by looking at the quantity of minerals, calories nutrients, and more. These can be compared to the food items that aid in reducing stress, or essential to live an active and healthy lifestyle. If you recognize that you're eating unhealthy foods which can cause stress, you are able to substitute the unhealthy foods with better ones.

It will also allow you determine if your eating habits were triggered by when you weren't hungry, or as a response to anxiety or mood fluctuations. The analysis will help you determine if you were over-eating or using the same kinds of meals over and over. If you have these information about your eating habits You can change the food items to adhere to a healthier eating plan.

An accurate food journal is vital since it can help to determine if you're doing the right thing. It can serve as a way to learn the foods that provide important nutrition to your diet, and which ones don't. It is then possible to utilize this knowledge to formulate your own healthy eating program that will lead you towards living a peaceful and healthy lifestyle free of tension.

Physical Exercise

For the week I, record every day in your journal regarding the quantity of programming as well as routine exercises you participated in. Programed exercises are like walking, swimming and attending a fitness center or the gym using an exercise bike or lifting weights. Regular exercise is what that you can get through your regular daily activities. It could be as simple as taking the stairs rather than an elevator or an escalator, or even park your car further from the door. This could also mean taking a bicycle for a ride to work or to the grocery store instead of driving.

A. Choose one or two areas that you could improve the exercise you have planned.

B. Give two suggestions on how you can enhance your routine fitness.

Stress Exercises

Which strategies did you employ this week to lessen the anxiety? Have you engaged in an practice like meditative and listening to soothing music or yoga, an entertaining film, practiced an exercise that required deep breathing, or and took a break from job? What peaceful activities have you engaged in over the last week? Make a list of at least three activities below.

1.

2.

3.

Week I Summary

After you've completed the research you've done After you have completed your research, it is time to summarise the results.

A. My DASS scores as well as the areas that I am concerned about are:

B. Four or three important points I learned through this week's Journal this week include:

A. A. Attitudes or beliefs I observed were_____.

b. The emotions I experienced frequently were those of _____.

C. Relationships that are positive or negative which I am in are _____.

D. D. My experience of behavior that I considered useful or damaging was _____.

C. Do I have to alter my diet as component of the Action Plan? What are three of the most significant things I have learned regarding my diet?

D. What I've learned this week about my workout practices?

E. What types of strategies for stress reduction have I found most useful this week?

Week II

Physical Exercise

We have mentioned in the previous chapters how exercise has many advantages for decreasing stress and increasing brain health, and so on.

In this week's session, you'll start introducing a fresh exercise program into your workout routine. In the following list, the exercise you're planning to choose?

Walking

When:

Where:

How Long:

Swimming

When:

Where:

How Long:

Running

When:

Where:

How Long:

This week, incorporate a fresh routine activity in your routine. Like, for example.

"I am planning to park my car just 100 yards from the front door of my work location and stroll. Once I am inside the building, I'll go up the elevator to the fourth floor and continue walking up the remaining two floors to get my workplace."

Record your routine on this page:

Week III

Stress Management Technique

In this week's time, implement a stress-management strategy to your routine. Choose an activity which is easy for you to complete and which you are enjoying. It is likely that you will remember from prior chapters that the actions include deep abdominal exercises, diaphragmatic bathing and mediation yoga, floatation, and meditation.

In the box below write down the activities you plan to include in your agenda this week.

When:

Where:

How Long:

Week IV

Nutrition/Supplementation

We'll be able to recall that eating well is essential for physical and mental well-being. Based on the information you gathered through our self-assessment during week 1, which two methods of managing your nutrition or supplements will be the most beneficial for you?

A.

B.

Week V

Thought Patterns

If you've been studying that the way we think can have a lot in determining our feelings and in the end, how we behave. Positive affirmations are a way to counteract negativity or negative beliefs that hinder our ability to reach our goals. They are also known as "limiting beliefs".

In your journal Do you spot some negative thought patterns? Did you realize you were putting yourself down? Are you putting pressure on the individuals you know? You were asking you "What if this or what if that or only if this or that would happen?" Do you feel that you found yourself focusing on the wrong issues that occurred throughout the week?

What thought patterns could I alter this week? What can I do to help me reduce my stress level?

In the example above, if I am tempted to say that they or I should... I'll alter my "should" into it would be more effective If they did...

What affirmations can you positively say to yourself in the coming week?

As an example, "Each and every day I am getting better in every way."

Chapter 7: The Importance of Optimum Mental Health in Today's World

A lot of emphasis is put on staying physically well-fit. There is no reason not to suggest that getting fit is now a trend and a trend

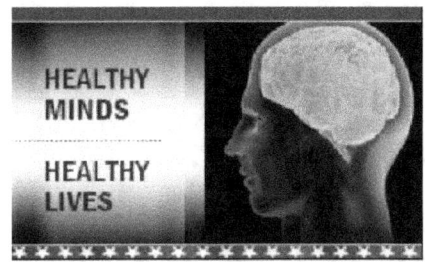

which people want to be a part of. That's why you'll observe people doing exercise as well as eating healthier food. But equally crucial is their mental wellbeing. If you are not in optimum mental health there's nothing that you could do, even as you're in excellent physical shape.

It is important to recognize the reality that it's the brain which controls the body and not in reverse. When your brain's functioning at its maximum capacity then you can't expect it to fulfill its duties properly. Furthermore, without optimal mental health, the level of happiness decreases, as does the risk of developing health issues grows.

The brain fog issue is only one of many mental health issues that you could be prone to over time. However, this is becoming more frequent these days. A healthy mind can help you to avoid these issues that affect the body and mind, and enjoy a fulfilling and happy life. Like you, it's not an idyllic paradise. There are numerous obstacles and obstacles to overcome on your journey.

Mental health is a top priority which will allow you to get over these challenges. If your mind isn't prepared to handle the challenges that life throws at you It becomes hard to overcome the challenges. A majority of those suffering from depression are the ones who haven't made the effort to enhance their mental health and discover a method of helping endure the rough moments in their lives.

In the current world of high-pressure the importance of maintaining a healthy mind is more crucial than ever before. If you don't have the brain capability to perform at the top at your job it is unlikely to be successful. It is because there is always someone waiting to succeed you just as fast after you have failed. Thus, you must remain strong physically and mentally to keep ahead of others who are competing for similar things the same way as you.

Additionally, there's an increasing concern by medical professionals that more and more individuals have been exhibiting anti-social behaviours. This is a lot to have to do with brain fog and the other mental issues that individuals have to face. It is difficult for them to connect regularly with those that surround them. This leads people to depression and isolation. Mentally strong is the best way to shield yourself from solitude.

Your mental health is directly influenced by your mental well-being. If your brain isn't healthy enough, it's nearly impossible to deal with your emotions. They remain locked within and trigger frustration and anguish, and for that there's no way to release them. The emotions often manifest with a way that is difficult to think of. Therefore, it is essential that you discover ways to stimulate your brain.

The best part is that the brain is actually a muscle. It is a fact that we often are often prone to overlook. As with any muscle that require exercise, the brain is no exception. As you work it, the more powerful it will become. It doesn't mean you have to devote hours at the gym to exercise. In the end, maintaining your mental well-being isn't nearly as hard when you work out to increase your physical health.

In light of the importance of optimal mental health today this is why it's more important that you strive toward improving your health.

What is Brain Fog?

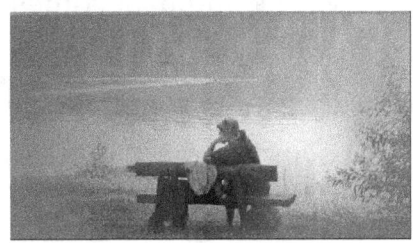

There is a good chance that you'll know the definition of fog and how it affects the surrounding. If there's fog, visibility diminishes and everything looks blurred. It is difficult to clearly see things even with your eyes in close proximity towards your eyes. The thicker the fog is more difficult it is to manage. The brain fog can be akin to this. It's like your mind is clouded. it isn't possible to utilize it in the way you usually do.

As per medical professionals, the word used for brain fog refers to "clouding of consciousness". If the person's conscious is unclear, the person has a problem with mental clarity. The mind becomes clouded and this causes a decrease in awareness. Brain fog, however, is not as serious as delirium. The symptoms are quite minor and do not appear physically obvious.

A loss of ability to be able to think clearly could render an individual powerless and ineffective. The result is a feeling of despair and depressed because the person isn't able to recall things, and attempts to separate himself from the rest of society. In contrast to other psychological disorders it doesn't come with "attacks" or "phases". It's generally speaking always a mental health condition that is able to get worse or better dependent on the way one is coping with the issue.

The biggest obstacle for diagnosis of brain fog is the fact the lack of a barometer by which an individual could be tested. Therefore, it's dependent and subject to interpretation. Anyone affected realizes they're struggling to think clearly, however, they are not likely to report it to a professional in mental health. It is the reason that the brain fog of dementia from anxiety, depression, etc.

There are a variety of variations on the process of brain fog that occurs within a person. In some cases, it can begin at a young time. As time passes the person begins to feel like this is their normal method of thinking. But for some the brain fog may increase as they getting older. The most common reason is if an individual is a victim of any of the common causes for the brain fog.

There is no age limit for brain fog, either. The condition can impact a toddler in the same manner it can affect a mature person.

However, adults have the ability to handle the issue in a way that children do not. The condition is very widespread, far more so than you would expect. This causes a myriad of problems for patients, such as problems with relationships, accidents and a lack of confidence in oneself that limit their potential throughout life.

The people suffering from brain fog tend to commit criminal acts or infractions that could have been avoided or had not. It is caused by struggles to connect with family members or friends. Feelings of loneliness and loneliness can result in at times a violent end. Therefore, it's essential to make more people aware of brain fog, and offered treatment when discovered to suffer from it.

Recognizing the root causes of cognitive fog can be a significant way to get started. In this way, you will determine if you stand the chance to succumb to the condition. Below are a few causes of your brain to appear to be as San Francisco does during the springtime.

Chapter 8: Causes of Brain Fog

Fatigue

Working too much and not getting enough sleep can lead to tiredness. If you feel tired constantly your body and mind aren't functioning properly. In many cases, absence of adequate sleep can lead to brain dysfunction that could lead people to think that they have some sort of mental health issue. Actually, you require enough sleep to tackle the issue and that's all it takes.

To achieve this, you'll be required to modify your sleep routine to some degree. In the beginning, it is essential that you are sleeping for 8 or 9 hours per evening. Additionally, you should try to unwind prior to going to go to bed. Do not work until late before going into bed immediately after. When you're at trying to avoid the consumption of coffee or other beverages that are caffeine-rich near the time you go to bed.

Stress

It is believed that stress is one of the primary cause of many ailments today, both physically and mentally. Stress may also lead to mental fog if you fail to discover a solution to ease the. The best way to reduce stress is to take a break on your work load and strive to make the most of your leisure time as you can. Stress can also trigger sensations of tiredness. Thus, it causes the two-pronged effects that can result in the brain becoming sluggish.

Stress is a problem in that it may stimulate your brain in a way that is not what normal. In the end, it becomes difficult for you to sleep and unwind effectively. Exercise is an excellent way to ease anxiety. Additionally, you can alter your diet and incorporating healthy diet. It's not only going to help you alleviate stress, but will improve your mood too.

Depression

Depression is the most common psychological condition in the US and more than 10% of the people being affected by it. Depression's effects include difficulties in focusing and remembering. Additionally, depression affects the capacity to take important decision. These are all results of brain fog too. Patients suffering from depression need to take steps to stop getting cognitive fog.

Chronic Fatigue Syndrome

Chronic fatigue syndrome can be attributed as a condition that weakens your brain's ability. In the event that your immune system isn't working well, it's likely that you will experience fatigue all day long. The best way to improve your magnesium levels for this issue. A light exercise routine can assist you to manage chronic fatigue syndrome.

Nutritional Deficiencies

There's a huge list of essential nutrients your brain requires in order to continue running at its best. It is important to note that your brain is the one that really focuses on these essential nutrients. Therefore, it is important to be sure that your supply is compatible with what you consume, otherwise it may result in nutritional deficiencies. If your brain doesn't get the nutrients it needs the brain is suffering from fog. It's just one of the many ailments which can develop.

Toxic Metals

Being in contact with harmful metals may increase the likelihood that a person will develop cognitive fog. There are many toxic metals associated with headaches, including copper. Copper imbalances inside the body may result in brain fog that it is difficult to determine. The factors listed above can be the direct cause of copper deficiency, as is the usage of birth medication to control it.

Trace Minerals

Together with the toxic metals excess levels of trace mineral within the body could cause mental fog. It is true that some of the minerals which can trigger this problem are that your body requires frequently like manganese and iron.

Mental Ailments

Because the brain is affected by a fog problem, it's normal that other mental illnesses can contribute to its development and progression throughout the body. The most frequent cause is the existence of brain parasites, which could create problems such as Lyme's Disease which can cause the inability of a brain to function.

Overstimulation

A few people are over exuberant. They have trouble controlling their own emotions and an overwhelming percentage of them have been diagnosed with Attention Deficit Disorder (ADD) that is among the signs that are a result of brain fog. The lack of a sense of balance could be the primary cause however, it's a condition that can be dealt with easily.

Drug Use

Pharmaceuticals, drugs as well as narcotics, may cause various mental issues including the brain becoming fogged. If your mind is affected by stimulants that cause hallucinations, it can be hard for the user to think rationally or clear. In the past, we have said that your brain's a muscle that requires regular exercises. The use of drugs actually hinders the exercising.

Hypoglycemia

The majority of people aren't conscious of the fact that blood sugar levels are low and could cause cognitive fog. This is due to the fact that the energy our brain needs comes from energy stored in your body. But, your brain can not keep the calories in its system and must receive these daily from the body. If your blood sugar levels decreases, the brain becomes not able to absorb the nutrients it needs for optimal functioning and this causes confusion in the brain.

They are a few of the frequent causes of the brain fog. However, they are not the only causes, so you must be cautious in your eating habits as well as the amount of activities you undertake during your day. A healthy diet and adequate rest is a sure way to ensure your brain is not affected by fog. The methods to get rid of brain fog further in this ebook.

You should already have an idea of the term "brain fog. Though it's not being a serious psychological issue however, it could create enough issues to your everyday life that might find difficult to handle. In the next section we'll explore the ways it can impact the different aspects of your life.

Chapter 9: How Brain Fog Affects Your Personal and Professional Life

It could appear to you that the effects of brain fog are only felt by the individual suffering from it. However, one can't ignore the impact of this condition on everyone around that person, specifically their relatives and acquaintances. They must bear all the burdens of this condition in order to assist the person get over the problem that

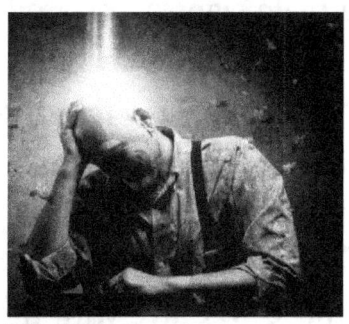

has been afflicting them.

Similar to any other mental health issue the brain fog can affect everything in your everyday life. It is difficult to focus as well as remember information and make the right choices. These can cause serious problems both at home and at workplace. In this manner, the brain fog can have an adverse effect on both your professional and personal life. We'll look at a few of the negative effects.

Effects on Personal Life

Short-Temperedness & Irritability

One of the main signs associated with brain fog is the individual affected is unhappy almost all of every day. They are irritable, and even any slight issue can cause a massive eruption of anger. Naturally, it can create problems within the family, especially those who live with their partner, spouse or children. If you're not able to be happy no matter the effort you put into it you will find it difficult to make friends with people who is around you.

A different issue is the irritability associated with this mental disorder. A person is constantly annoyed regardless of the actual reason behind it. Sometimes, this can result in a violent display and can lead to further issues. Even though the family of the victim may feel the desire to be there for them, different relationships including colleagues, friends and family can also be affected.

Irrational Thinking

If you've lost the ability to focus A person who suffers of brain fog is unable to be trusted to take major decisions. It is a huge hit to their self-confidence because there's not much they can do to restore the lost confidence. As time passes, they begin finding that they are trusted less with big responsibilities as well as decisions. This further lowers confidence in themselves.

Additionally, it can lead to an irrational way of thinking and behaviour. People start to have shady thoughts that could lead to issues for him/her. As the mind becomes affected by the illness and the person is unable to make any rational decisions, they are able to accomplish to convince themselves that they believe otherwise.

Trust Issues

Problems with trust are often a result from brain fog. Like we said, the reduced thinking ability of the individual causes others to believe less and less in them. In addition those who suffer from mental fog is also prone to doubts in their mind regarding their surroundings. This could cause problems in the event that these fears come to light.

It can be difficult for anyone to convince someone to let go of any questions they are pondering in their head. Because they lack an means to get rid of those doubts they remain in their hearts and thoughts, which causes a decline in the mental state of their patients. Brain fog increases and it is extremely difficult to recover from it over the long term.

Constant Frustration

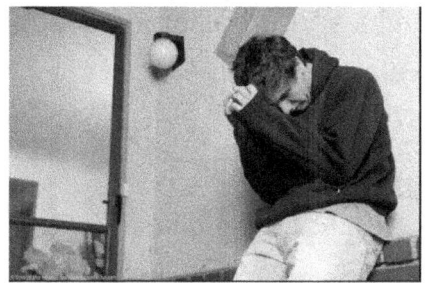

It is becoming increasingly difficult to control the feeling of anger in your body when you struggle with the fog of your mind. It is more likely to be due to your inability to utilize your brain to the fullest extent than being a sign that you suffer from an illness of the mind. A growing sense of frustration can lead to stress and anger that usually is manifested in an antisocial attitude.

This is not only a source of displeasure for the patient, but to the others around them. As they observe the lack of motivation as well as worsening mental state firsthand, they begin losing hope. Then they begin to feel dissatisfied that an individual with talent might end up using their abilities due to a curable mental illness.

Stigma

In spite of all the advances in the field of medicine and acceptance of mental illnesses however, these disorders remain by many as being stigmatized. If you suffer with mental fog, the situation differs as, more often than not, it isn't diagnosed. The patient must take care of themselves without assistance from medical professionals.

It is one of the main reasons for the sufferer of the condition of brain fog often spends their time sitting in their rooms or at home, because they cannot accept the rejection and sympathy shown to them by others. There isn't a method to escape this, but there's no evidence that this has an impact directly on both the personal and professional life of someone who suffers from brain fog.

Here are a few ways that cognitive fog impacts your daily life. It is evident that a few aspects of this can affect the professional side of your life. There are a few issues that relate to the professional world and the effects that the brain fog can have on your life.

Effects on Professional Life

Fatigue and Exhaustion

In the preceding section, the condition of brain fog is often accompanied by exhaustion and fatigue. The cause is clear enough: the individual's brain is engaged by some thing or other. The stress is too high on the mind, and it is impossible to allow it to rest. When one is constantly tired and exhausted every day is it difficult to achieve the best of.

This can have a significant effect on the productivity of a person on the job. In addition to the fact that the same issue could be a problem in the home, the consequences can be more severe in relation to their work. They're not able to exert the energy required to keep their

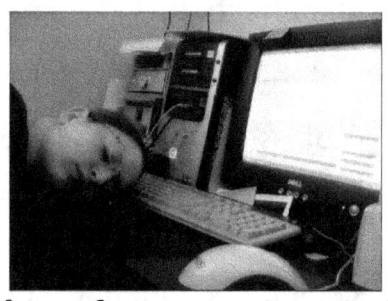

graph of performance in good shape. Additionally, it's hard for them to work too much, which may cause subpar or ineffective job.

It's not just a matter of affecting confidence in themselves, but it also affects the likelihood of success at the job. Employment growth standards depend more or less around the quality and quantity of work that a worker can perform. This ability can be impaired significantly, and it is unlikely that people suffering from brain fog will have the ability to excel in their professional career.

Chapter 10: The Work Environment

The negative effects of brain fog in the professional world aren't just restricted to the performance of your employees. No doubt, your relationship with your superiors and colleagues can affect the quality of your work. As a result of cognitive fog, you'll have a difficult time being respectful with your coworkers. It could become more sensitive when the person who suffers of brain fog gets unjustly treated.

If that happens the situation is a bit difficult to stop the person from doing something. The person will not only be very angry, but they may also have a difficult time trying to perform at that level later on. As their brain isn't in a state of mind the way they think, they'll perceive this as a retribution to them. As time passes, this can cause further problems with colleagues and supervisors.

Handling Responsibility

There's a distinction in the way you handle the responsibility of home as opposed to work. In your home, you're not being assessed on how well you manage the burden. However, at work this could be the factor that determines the success or failure of your career based on how you manage the situation. However, the issue is that you may not get a job in the first place due to the psychological issue.

As hard as you try but it's hard to convince people that you are able to manage difficult situations and take good choices all the times. The result is that you are overlooked for possibilities that would otherwise be in your hands. Again, there's nothing you can do about it, other than trying to get rid of the mental fog.

Impaired Memory

The last but certainly not last, but certainly not last, but certainly not the least, brain fog affects the way you remember things. It's difficult for you to recall events that have taken place in the past. This makes it more likely for you to losing things that are essential, for example your work that you must finish in the course of a time or the meeting you're supposed to be attending. It will be difficult to perform and productive at work.

In the meantime this will also have an influence on your personal relationship and life. The tendency to lose track of small details that can cause huge disagreements as well as friction with those in your circle of social friends. You can't effectively do to ensure that you do not forget crucial things as your brain is enclosed by the cloud of brain.

When compared to the issues mentioned previously, memory loss may not appear like a huge problem, but it can be. It is evident when you experience brain fog that makes your memory shaky. You may not remember the day your children were born or the exact date when you meet with a key customer.

You can now see the personal and professional life is in jeopardy when you begin to experience mental fog. It's up to you to discover a solution to your issue. To get you started in the right direction We have offered some suggestions for clearing your brain fog. They will be discussed in the next section.

Diagnosing Brain Fog

The primary concern that psychology specialists have about brain fog is the difficulty of the condition. There's no specific diagnostic test that can be utilized to determine the cause as well as there's no prescribed criteria a doctor must follow when a patient exhibits one of the signs related to the condition.

But, at the exact at the same time, it's crucial that an accurate analysis is conducted of the patient's symptoms to identify the severity of the issue. If they have more signs and the more intense the first are, the higher the possibility of having the condition known as brain fog. Family members or yourself are advised to look out for the common signs like difficulties with attention, forgetfulness as well as disorientation.

Another thing that doctors are able to perform is test patients for the factors that cause headaches. In the case of patients have been exposed to harmful metals frequently this could indicate that they're suffering from this illness. A patient who follows an omnivore diet may experience the condition of brain fog.

This is that it is ideal for specialists within the field to join together for figuring out the best way to accurately diagnose cognitive fog. Unfortunately, the condition hasn't been recognized as a mental illness up to the present. In the meantime, until attitudes towards the condition changes, it's hard to believe that a cure will be found.

Tips for Clearing the Brain Fog

The only way to eliminate your brain fog is by regaining control over your thinking and allowing it to do what it was designed to. Most sufferers give in to the brain fog, and fail to discover a solution to conquer it. In time, their situation gets worse until there's no cure for their condition.

However, there are ways to get rid of the mental cloud that has been engulfing your brain.

Regain Your Focus

First, you must get back on track. This is much more challenging than you think. It is important to remember the things you'd like to accomplish in your the world. If your brain is cluttered and you're not thinking clearly It is very possible to get lost in your objectives. Therefore, the most important thing to be reminded of which your life's goals are. Although it may not affect your life immediately, but it is a crucial move.

One reason for finding it difficult to focus is because your brain is working too hard. What you must discover is a method for it to calm. When you are suffering from the fog of your brain, it's difficult to relax. However, there must be some thing that can make you feel relaxed and calm. This could be walking in the park, or performing a piano. Whatever the case it is, you must locate it and get started with it. It'll lead to getting back on track.

Boost Your Concentration

In addition to your concentration is concentration, which is a crucial aspect. If you're not able to focus on the most important issues in your life, the odds that your life will become out of hand within a matter of minutes. The second factor to improve your focus is to improve your concentration. It is true that this could be more challenging than getting your focus back. The reason is the fact that your attention is built upon your objectives, which are rooted in the mind of your. Focusing is an entirely different thing

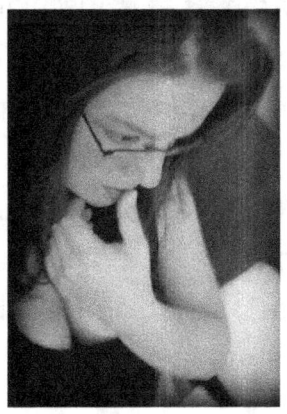

entirely.

There are numerous exercises that you can do to increase your focus. These are games for the mind that allow you to concentrate more than ever before. Try the art of meditation. It has two benefits. It improves your concentration while at the same time assist you in staying focused throughout your life. Find an opportunity to include mindfulness into your your daily life.

Increase Your Attention Span

Reiterating a statement I mentioned before that your brain is a muscular organ and requires exercising. Your attention span is just one of many things that depend on how much exercise your brain gets each day. The more you work your mind, the greater your focus will improve. The ability to focus has an immediate impact on the ability of your mind to concentrate and focus.

The act of reading, solving problems and studying or just being able to think can enhance your concentration significantly. This is something you need to strive for. The more adept you are to concentrate is, the simpler it is easier to manage your mind confusion.

Chapter 11: Learn to Think Straight

Perhaps this is the most vital aspect of your entire effort to eliminate your brain fog. The most obvious effect of the brain fog affects your ability to focus. There must be ways to do this or else you'll not have the ability to eliminate the fog in your brain. First thing to accomplish in this area is begin physical activity. It's not just only for a few days. It is essential to make exercising an ongoing part of your day and element of your routine.

Naturally, you do not need to work out each day. In the end, you're getting rid of brain fog and rather than building muscles. In order to get back to your original goal it is possible to adhere to a brief and easy regimen. It should focus on your capacity to stick to your routine every day. That's why the simpler it gets, the better for your health. The only thing you need to do is spend thirty minutes every day, every single day of the week working out in order for a chance to focus.

For a better chance to be successful, it's recommended to begin working out outside. A fresh breeze and sun will help to alleviate your emotional and mood issues for a considerable amount. With the efforts that you make to increase the focus, concentration and concentration exercising will help the mind to be clear. Once you've mastered this clearing your brain of the fog will be simple.

Improve Your Memory

Also, you must focus on your memory, and figure out an approach to increase the quality of it. In the absence of this, you do not stand a possibility of being able to eliminate the fog in your head. Your memory depends on your ability to pay attention as well as your ability to focus. When you've dealt with the two of them, you're likely to enhance your memory.

The most effective way to boost your memory is to continue doing exercises. The evidence suggests that doing exercises is a fantastic method to get rid of cloud of memory. If you're regularly exercising frequently the chances of having brain fog are reduced significantly.

Release Mental Stress

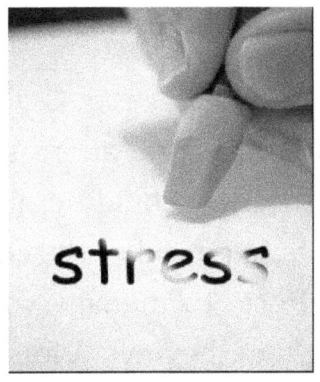

Relaxing your mind is just similar to breathing. Do not underestimate the effect stress has on your mental wellbeing. It's believed as the primary reason behind the majority of physical and mental disorders in the present. Therefore, there's nothing you can do to escape the stress that you're dealing with.

Exercise will definitely help relieve stress. Additionally it is also important to eat a healthy eating plan and have regular rest. If you're more relaxed at ease, the less stressed you'll be. Therefore, it is important to eliminate the stress that you feel experiencing.

If you see a physician to address your issues with headache, you could be given a range of treatments to get rid of the issue. Making your own efforts to manage your illness is an excellent idea however, you will require professional assistance in the event of. There is no way to know when symptoms become more severe and you're incapable of handling the situation.

A few tests are necessary prior to a physician being certain that you suffer from this problem. The doctor may ask you to undergo an MRI or CT scan prior to starting the treatment. They may also inquire regarding any conditions or allergies that you may have to establish if you will get the typical treatment.

It is then that the treatment began in full force. In this phase you'll need to take a variety of medications, pills or herbs, vitamins and minerals and occasionally hormones. The type of supplements you take depends on the root of the issue. That's why the treatments for brain fog will vary from one individual to another. There's not a universal remedy and your physician will recommend an appropriate treatment based on the medical condition and signs.

Before ending, it's essential to identify something. One of the main causes of cognitive fog and its numerous signs is a poor diet. If you're not eating sufficient healthy meals you will experience an effect on your brain. The brain requires nutrients that must be provided. Modifying your diet to make it healthier can help eliminate mental fog.

Chapter 12: Brain Power Food

Once I understood the condition I was in, what I discovered was that my low energy was not caused by my learning difficulties, but was because of the routines I'd developed through my entire life. The habits began to develop in my attempt to deal with the challenges I was facing but, as time passed they became more pronounced and added to my list problems.

My first thing I'd like to pay attention to is the way we eat. For me, over most of my life food was the food source of comfort. I was always anxious, depressed and frightened. I felt at ease eating sweet, rich fat, sugary and salty food items. They tasted delicious, and they felt good. At the time I did not see that as a terribly bad choice. Giving myself treats was my method of taking care for my self. If I felt depressed or angry, I longed like I needed ice cream, or the such. In addition the fact that my understanding of managing my time was low. It was a constant struggle to be up by the time I needed so I was always being over my time. Breakfasts for me were usually quick, typically toast, or the occasional cup of coffee.

The most important things I've learned was that the old adage was "What you put in is what you get out." I was averse to this phrase because I often believed that I did my very best but I wasn't getting results. When I heard that I felt as if people said that I wasn't doing my best. In all honesty I still don't like the meaning of that phrase but I would rather look at it more figuratively. What we put into our bodies directly impacts the results we receive from us. By understanding the way food impacts the brain and body, we'll begin to realize how crucial eating healthy can be for transforming the way you live and unleashing the full potential of you.

The chapter's title does not mean just food, but the power of your brain. Right now while you're in the process of reading or listening to the article Your brain is in good shape. It's processing the sounds of your eardrums as well as the light that is in your eyes, and determining significance from the information. Every thought that you make and every move you make is determined by the brain. Arm raise, then tighten your fist. Get up and take an extra step. Move your head left side, and then the right. Everything was accomplished by the brain. Our brain regulates the body, our mood, emotions as well as many other things.

This book focuses on three aspects: ways to lift yourself out from brain fog the best way you can unlock your maximum potential, and the best way to enhance your brain's abilities. Before we can explore ways to increase the power of our brain it is essential to determine the fundamentals of where our brain's power originates. Brains are only about two percent of our bodies in average, but it accounts for approximately

20 percent of our use of energy (Altomare and co. 2017, 2017).

What is the definition of energy? In physics, the term "energy" is described as the ability to perform work. For our purposes, energy is the thing that is supplying our bodies, and in particular our brains, all entire day. Your body's cells are constantly producing energy, even when we sleep. In order to keep our brains working optimally, it is essential to maintain the level of energy we have.

How does this apply to our food choices and food we consume? In the first place it is important to know that humans generate energy is through drinking of beverages and food. If we were batteries and we were a battery, the only way to be charged would be through food. The amount and quality of charge we're getting is derived from the food and drinks that we consume daily and eat, also which is known as our diet.

Let's start with the initial essential step towards increasing your brain's power which is to ensure that your body is fueled with the fuel and nutrition necessary to perform at its maximum potential.

Caloric Intake

In keeping with the metaphor of quality and quantity of the product We'll start by looking at the aspect of 'quantity. The quantity, in comparison to the quality will be more comprehensible. It's all about the amount we consume and the reason we ought to be mindful of our eating habits. This means not consuming too much, however, you shouldn't starve your body. If you've ever attempted to shed weight, then you've probably been told in order to "watch your calories." You may have friends who appear to eat whatever they'd like and don't gain weight and then you wonder what the reasons are. One reason is that it is the concept that you are "watching your calories."

What exactly is an Calories? If we are talking about the energy that is associated with our body and food, we employ a particular measuring unit called the calories. This is precisely what the calories is. It's a means to quantify the amount of the energy that food can provide us after consumption. Additionally, it can be used to indicate how much energy burned in physical exercise.

Calories are all over the place in the world of food items. In the case of buying food items from food stores, the quantity of calories in them will always be mentioned on the back of the package in the nutrition information typically the first item on the listing. These numbers don't mean anything in the absence of a fundamental understanding about what they are.

A mile of walking can, in the average, generate around 100 calories. Contrast that with eating an ordinary egg boiled will provide you with about 70 calories. Exercises that are strenuous and intense will use up more calories. In the same way, eating high-calorie in fatty, fat-rich foods with greater calories will provide your body with power and therefore lots of calories.

How Much Should I Eat?

If you're like me, and you want to comprehend something, you must to be aware of every aspect. It is my responsibility to silence the little voices that ask questions. One of the first concerns I was asked was, if food is a source of calories which are energy-rich then why don't I consume as much food as possible? It was answered quickly with just a few minutes of research on the dangers of excessive eating and obesity, heart disease as well as other conditions. It left me with a difficult question: how much I supposed to consume?

Food until satisfied is likely to be the most natural way to go. When you look into the realm of calories, the picture becomes somewhat unclear. Certain foods are loaded with energy and provide the body with hundreds of calories, but in a tiny amount. Some foods are low in calories yet are extremely full of calories. A lot of diets consist of foods that are low in calories and filling that give the feeling that you are fuller and consume less calories.

It is still a while before I address the issue of what amount of food you're supposed to eat. The reason for that is due to the fact that it's an extremely complex topic. The optimal daily caloric intake depends on the particulars of an particular person's metabolic rate, age, degree of physical exercise, as well as numerous different factors. In the end that, the recommended daily caloric intake should be around 2500 calories for women and 2500 calories for males. This is based upon the daily average of calories consumed and can be considered an estimate. To know more how much you need to eat it is recommended to speak with a doctor.

Weight Loss

What is so vital? The reason lies in the fact that all of these elements is interconnected. It is a simple fact that when your consumption of calories is higher the day than the body can burn and stores excess fat to use later. The body's fat stores are used for energy storage. This is the reason why "counting calories" stems from and the reason why, in diets designed to lose weight it is important to track your intake of calories to ensure that you consume less calories than the body requires. You will be left with an energy shortage that in essence the body will be forced to use its stored excess of energy. In other words, it will have to burn off some of the stored of body fat in order to replenish the energy.

If you're looking to shed weight with an eating plan, you should exercise caution regarding the program you're adhering to. You should get advice from a dietetic professional instead of using one of the numerous thirty-day weight loss plans available that are available online. In the past, we have discussed how eating less calories can help in losing weight due to the body's ability to burn fat stores. The greater the deficit in calories, more fat needs to be burnt to cover the deficit. A lot of the overly strict diets go too far, and recommend extremely limited food intake that could be harmful to the health of your body.

You should eat a balanced diet to maintain good brain health. When it comes to overeating, undereating and eating with moderate amounts, it is best to aim towards the last. In the trio, undereating is the most harmful as is a deficiency of food is among the most life-threatening.

Starvation

If we aren't able to provide the required energy by eating food, our body's first priority is to eat its fat reserves or reserves, which can have the effect of leading us to shed weight. But what happens when these reserves start to deplete? As reserves get extremely low, our body starts to consume away at muscle tissue, which causes the body to weaken. The process is referred to as hunger. What is the reason it's important to understand this? because we must be aware that our body is wired and designed to be able to survive at any cost. The basic human instincts we have are designed to survive, and our bodies have developed numerous mechanisms throughout time that have helped to ensure. The most notable method I'm going to talk about below is what the body is doing when it's constantly being pushed to consume the energy reserves it has, and decrease the speed at which it is burning.

Metabolic Rate

The metabolic rate refers to the rate at which your body uses energy throughout the course of. When this rate is reduced it slows the rate it converts energy. Through reducing the pace of which it needs to devour the energy reserves and extending its time frame before it's going to have to consume of its muscle tissue. The balance helps us avoid hunger, but this isn't always easy. If we are aware that due to a an accelerated metabolic rate we'll be producing lesser energy over the course of time How can be drawn?

It is the energy that drives each and every decision If we do not have enough in energy generation, we'll certainly be exhausted. There will be a feeling of a low energy and often you may feel exhausted and lethargic. If we experience that, it becomes difficult to stay focused and achieve the highest level.

Semi-Starvation

It is possible to ask how come we're discussing hunger? For us or at least mine it was a phenomenon that was only experienced in extreme cases due to a long-term lack of food. How is this relevant? It was interesting to realize that my perception of hunger was foolish. There is no switch that flips after a long period of time in a famine. There are a variety of events, one of which slows our metabolism rate. It is caused by our body in times of absence of food. It is triggered by skipped meals, skipped breakfasts and, most importantly losing weight diets.

A long-term habit of eating may affect the rate of metabolic change that we experience over time. This is the reason it's crucial, regardless of whether you are trying to lose weight to make sure you're having regular meals, and taking in sufficient calories to help you get through your daily. How much fuel your body receives directly determines the amount of tasks you're able to do this is why I am going to the next tip.

The Importance of Breakfast

Sometimes in the event that I ran over my time, mainly because of my inability of waking up in time, I'd try cut down on breakfast. On some days, I could have had toast for a piece and a cup or coffee or even nothing whatsoever. I suffered from these symptoms that I was overwhelmed, anxious and depressed about my work, unable to relax and focus from my surroundings, and often irritable. Although I now know that the majority of them are due to my disabilities in learning however, I wasn't helping any of the issues in skipping breakfast. actually, I was creating a worse situation for myself.

Of all the food choices you'll have throughout the day, breakfast is considered to be the most crucial. If we're sleeping it isn't a time to eat and yet our bodies continue to burn fuel. In the hours when we're asleep but taking a break from eating, we're basically eating a fast. Breakfast is essentially a way to break the fast' and get your energy back to start the day. It is essential to have that energy in order to keep us going and start your day in a healthy way.

Make sure you're providing your brain with the right nutrients. I've made it clear before however it is worth not being forgotten. The brain is the controller of every part of your body from breathing to the beat of your heart. Consuming enough food and following an appropriate, balanced diet will ensure that your brain gets the necessary sources of energy and the resources needed for functioning at maximum potential.

Nutrition

Although brief, we've discussed the basic quantity element of our diets. We now move on to one of the most important aspects of twoaspects, which is quality. When I say quality refers to the nutritional value of the food we consume. In addition to the energy the food we eat contain a wide array of nutrients are essential for our bodies for proper functioning. In this post I will explain the various nutrients that we need and where they come from, and the functions they are used for. When you understand this it will help you to comprehend the advantages as well as the importance of healthy eating habits.

While the initial thing to do is that you're eating enough of the food you need to supply your body's needs for energy however, it isn't enough to constitute a nutritious eating plan. A healthy lifestyle is more than just taking in enough calories daily. It's about mixing up your choices of what that you consume and keeping in balance the various food categories.

What is the reason we need an additional amount of food? What is the reason we can't eat the food we love every all day long, at every meal? Our food choices breakdown into the energy as well as nutrients within the body. Certain foods break down in different ways and are converted into various substances. The body requires a constant intake different vitamins, nutrients, and minerals to function optimally. When it comes to studying the subject of nutrition in relation to diet and body and the body, attention is split into two categories that are macronutrients as well as micronutrients.

Macronutrients

To make this publication, we will briefly discuss macronutrients. This word might sound intimidating however, if you look at it in a different way into smaller pieces, the concept is easy. The word macro means "at a large scale," therefore, for this instance, macronutrients will be the primary or most significant portion of the ingredients found in our diets. Three macronutrients are:

Carbohydrates

The term is often used to refer to them as carbs. carbohydrates make up a significant portion of a variety of diets. When eating healthy they will constitute the majority of everyday energy that we need because they're disintegrated and absorbed. Carbohydrates constitute the primary energy source of the body because they are broken down into energy much faster than fats. If you're in need of energy, and you need it fast carbs are your ideal all-rounder. Breakfasts that are a majority should consist of sugars.

Examples of carbohydrates are rice, bread and other grains.

Proteins

The muscles enable us to walk and move as well, and proteins are crucial in maintaining an overall healthy body. This is why proteins rarely get used into energy because their function in the care of muscles is crucial to our bodies. In this regard, you'll easily see why eating just one big steak at breakfast, although delicious and satisfying, it will be unable to provide the kind of energy to get through the day.

Some examples of protein sources are meat, chicken as well as poultry.

Fats

Fats have the highest energetic of all three. Fats are among the factors to consider in your efforts to shed weight. Because of their high content of calories, even tiny amounts of fat can significantly raise your daily intake of calories. Fats can be a great source for energy, however they aren't the first preference to consume.

They must be first transformed into fatty acids prior to when they can be converted into energy. When your body is in need of energy, it tends to use up carbs instead of. Since fats don't get used up in the normal course of existence, they'll be stored and later used in the body. That is the reason why a diet that is loaded with fats can lead to weight increase. It is tempting to attempt to cut out the fats from your diet, but do not. Fats are still a crucial element of a balanced diet as long as they're consumed in moderate amounts. They do begin to be burnt during long durations of exercise, like swimming, running or cycling.

Some examples of fats are oils and butter.

Ratio

There's no definitive "golden" amount of each category should consume within their diet. In general, to have a balanced eating plan, it is somewhere between forty and sixty percent of your food intake from carbohydrates, 20 to 35 percent from fats while the remainder 10% to 35% comes from protein. The ratios depend upon the person and their degree of exercise throughout the entire day.

If you live an active lifestyle, and you engage in routine exercise, including exercise for strength, the quantity of protein you require is likely to increase. In contrast, if you live a more sedentary lifestyle, when your muscles do not have to endure the same strain as they are during regular exercise it is expected that the amount of protein you require will decrease.

Carbohydrates must always comprise most of the three as they're your primary energy source throughout your whole day. If you're not getting sufficient carbohydrates, you'll generally feel tired when the day progresses.

The presence of fats is a must in your food, but should not be the primary priority. It is important to consume them moderately. Keep in mind that fats have a high energy density by nature which makes it easy to eat too much and gain weight if you are consuming excessive amounts of fats in your food plan.

Building a Healthy Diet

There has been a lot of discussion about the importance of a balanced diet. But what exactly can be considered to be a healthy and balanced diet? A healthy diet encompasses many different types of food and is balanced. It is about eating enough calories to provide you with energy for your day-to-day needs without overindulging or eating too much with one food group.

However, a healthy nutrition is more than just how much foods you consume. The body demands more than just calories. There are essential nutrients present in food which our bodies require for proper functioning. A majority of these minerals, vitamins and minerals are readily available through beverages and food since the body is unable to synthesize these substances.

Insufficient nutrition can cause problems with a host of symptoms and may lead to more risky diseases. In order to ensure that we have an adequate supply of nutrients is only possible through eating a balanced, healthy diet. It is evident that each food group does not contain each mineral or vitamin needed by our bodies. Certain vitamins and minerals can be found in every food but some can only be found in meats, others in the fruits and vegetables while others are found in nuts as well as legumes.

Controlling your diet is among of the most important steps you do to transform your life. Foods you consume along with the nutrients you're not getting or consuming affect your body's functioning. Sometimes, the symptoms of deficiency are not severe like feelings of fatigue and tiredness, that can be attributed to another issue, not realizing that the cause is due to the food we eat.

It is common for us to treat the symptoms by drinking coffee in order to increase our energy levels as we're tired but do not manage to tackle the root of the problem, for instance an insufficient intake of carbs and vitamins.

Whatever your opinion, whether that your food habits are healthy for you, continue to look for ways to alter what you consume and make improvements to your eating habits. Consider adding more green leafy vegetables like spinach to your diet. Switch out potato chips for nutritious nuts, such as peanuts, almonds, or walnuts. Be sure to eat your meals regularly, and especially breakfast. Start your day with a cup of cup of coffee and some toast may not be enough of a meal to sustain you through the entire day.

What exactly is the best way to begin to change our food habits? Let's look at the example of widely-known and nutritious diet.

Mediterranean Diet

The Mediterranean diet has been believed to be among the healthiest food choices. In fact, for the past three consecutive years it has been awarded the title of being the most healthy general diet available in the US in accordance with the U.S. News & World Report annual ranking (Doheny 2020). The way of eating which focuses on vegetables and not animal products is in use since the beginning of time but the fascination with the benefits to health of this particular diet was first noticed in the 60s following the discovery that coronary heart disease was the cause of more deaths in Mediterranean nations, like Greece and Italy more than the US as well as northern Europe (Mayo Clinic Staff, 2019,).

The Mediterranean diet does not have an exact meal schedule however, it's the cuisine and food habits of countries that border the Mediterranean sea such as Morocco, Greece, and Italy. Contrary to most Western eating habits that place emphasis on meat particularly red meats and red meats, it is a Mediterranean diet is a plant-based. One of the main differences with this Mediterranean diet is its emphasis on vegetables and not meat as most meals include an abundance of fruit or other vegetables. Whole grains are the most popular. They are often substituted for white breads with whole grain varieties that also contain whole-grain varieties of cereal, rice and pasta.

Most people will use salt in their meals for flavor but within the Mediterranean diet spice and herbs are typically used in lieu, to amazing effect in creating flavor in the food.

The consumption of red meat is seldom, or only in tiny quantities. It is substituted with chicken, legumes, or more often than fish. Fish, as you may recall from the past, contains a lot of the essential nutrients that we need and are an ideal alternative to a more healthy choice of meat. It also contains dairy products specifically in the form of yogurts, cheeses and other dairy products.

Fats that are healthy, unprocessed and unsaturated constitute one of the key factors of diet. It is widely known that olive oil is the main fat consumed. Instead of cooking with butter or lard which is saturated fats, olive oil can be employed as a more healthy alternative. The seeds and nuts are essential sources of fats within your diet. In addition, the majority of Mediterranean food items are accompanied by wine, and are enjoyed by close friends and family.

Why Is the Mediterranean Diet so Healthy?

The majority of the time, it's observed that Western diets put too much emphasis on meat and forget that meat isn't the all-purpose food item. Our diets often contain excessive amounts of fat or protein particularly the bad type, saturated fats (found in fried food items as well as fatty pieces in red beef). These are fats that could negatively impact the health of our bodies and also affect the functioning of our body.

Though fats are vital to our bodies, excessive consumption of saturated fats including butter, lard, or the consumption of fatty meats is considered harmful since they can increase cholesterol levels and can cause strokes or coronary illnesses.

The Mediterranean diet is heavily based on fats. However, it is primarily healthy, unsaturated fats derived from seeds, nuts, as well as olive oil. The Mediterranean diet is rich in protein, not just from meat, but also dairy, legumes and even plants. Instead of red meat less fatty cuts of chicken as well as fish are preferred.

On most dishes there is a proportion of plant to meat tends to favor the vegetable. Fruits and vegetables make up the main ingredients of this meal and are delectable. It is often difficult to incorporate adequate amounts of fruits and vegetables into our diets due to adding the fruits and vegetables as an afterthought, but did not think about learning new recipes that highlight and highlight their finest qualities.

Alternative Diets

However, in spite of all benefits associated with it being a Mediterranean diet, it's not the only healthful diet that is available. It may not be the ideal food for everyone. The reason why the Mediterranean diet was designed here is because it's generalized, and it is more of a alteration in food habits.

There aren't any strict menu plans that you have to follow, and most crucially, there aren't any calories to track. A healthy diet that is suitable for each person is dependent upon a number of variables like weight, age the height, gender allergies and other preexisting ailments. The most effective way to find the diet best suited to your needs is to seek an expert medical opinion from a dietician trained to customize a food and diet plan specifically specific to your requirements. Naturally, this method does not work for all but it could be simpler to locate an online diet plan that you can adhere to. When this happens, cautiousness is suggested. Look for clinically reviewed menu programs.

These are a few final points to remember, regardless of the type of lifestyle you're on. The first is to ensure that you're eating a sufficient amount of food. Remember that, even if the objective is weight loss massive caloric deficiency in a continuous manner are a serious risk to health including semi-starvation which decreases your metabolism. In addition to the adverse effects and signs having a slower metabolic rate is also a slowing of the pace that you shed weight since your body will burn calories at a slower rate. Additionally, you should consider the macronutrient ratio.

Carbohydrates are the primary energy source, and they should make up the main component of your food intake. If you're seeking to gain muscle mass, don't overindulge in protein and do not forget to eat carbs. Be aware of your intake of fats, and try eating more healthy fats that lower cholesterol levels.

Also, remember the different minerals and vitamins that the body requires. Make sure that your menus comprise foods from every food category that will supply you with the essential nutrients that you need to be functioning properly. Don't forget the importance of legumes, vegetables as well as fruits and grains!

Allergies

Food allergies and other dietary restrictions may restrict the types of food you can consume, but there are many substitutes and alternatives that replace them. As an aside, I've observed a shift in my body's response to gluten. Even though I'm still able to eat gluten, in recent times I've noticed it's making my stomach hurt and cause constipation. For this reason I've tried to cut down on the gluten-based products from my diet. Because of this it has forced me to begin gradual replacing my mainstays by gluten-free choices.

Our bodies are always growing and evolving, and might develop intolerances or allergies to specific foods including dairy, gluten or nuts later in lives. The diet we follow are not established in stone. We should update them according in accordance with our changing circumstances.

Good Gut Health

I've come to enjoy food and am a fan of it which is why I'm always testing new meals and experiments on new dishes. Although I do occasionally indulge with a meal out, the method by how I pick new meals to incorporate into my meals since I cook my own food depends on a variety of aspects, such as diet, calories, food allergies and availability. I prefer to purchase fresh produce and seasonal vegetables whenever feasible. Most importantly, I like easy to digest foods that can be gentle on my digestive tract as they are essential for our mental and physical wellbeing. Actually, they're frequently referred to as our body's "second brain."

A number of studies indicate that the microbiome of our gut and our gut health has a significant part to play in controlling and preventing many different illnesses, primarily ones that affect the gut like irritable bowel syndrome and other conditions that impact the autoimmune and cardiovascular systems in the body. The possible role played by the gut's health on our mood and behaviour is demonstrated in several research studies (Ochoa-Reparaz and Kasper in 2016).

It is a belief that I firmly am convinced of. It's extremely difficult to concentrate with stomach issues. I was a bad time management, and I didn't cook any meals at home. Foods I consumed included take-outs and fast food. The spicy, fat, greasy and acidic foods have a negative impact on the intestinal tracts. The process of digesting these food items isn't simple for us, and it's not uncommon to experience nausea, bloating or irritable. as a result of an upset stomach.

After I started making my own meals, and was able to learn the foods that I must stay away from, my symptoms began to diminish. The result was a huge improvement in my mood. If you've required to stay in classes or have an upset stomach or work when you're nauseated, you're aware of how difficult to pay attention to any other thing than the stomach.

For this reason I aim to follow the right diet, which is kind for my stomach, and also improves my immune system. It is important to limit the amount of food I consume or take my food too fast so as not to place a strain on my stomach. I've eliminated coffee, and favor herbal teas with a light flavor. If you're a fan of coffee, that's okay, but be careful to avoid overdoing it. The effects of too much caffeine are harmful to the body, particularly the digestive system. If you notice abdominal pains or feeling nauseated after drinking your third or 4th drink of coffee, then it might be time to reduce your intake some.

Multivitamins & Supplements

An enlightened, diverse diet is the ideal approach, however it's important to realize that it may not be achievable for every person. Certain circumstances, including food allergies, as well as the accessibility and price of food could limit the food which we are able to get access to.

We are all fortunate to be living in an environment where supplements and multivitamins are able to fill in the gaps of our daily diet. An investigation conducted in

2014 on how to address deficiencies in nutrition with multivitamins and mineral supplements, which was published in Nutrition Journal, revealed that although these supplements are not able to be a substitute for consuming adequate quantities of diverse food items, they can help people who suffer from poor nutrition due to various causes. It was found to be a lack of all groups of food, advanced health, or chronic illnesses (Ward 2014.).

Despite my new diet There are minerals and vitamins I'm deficient in because of food shortages the place I reside, in addition to the allergies I have which is why I use supplements. I prefer taking supplements in the morning, after having breakfast. The majority of supplements should only be consumed after eating as they're more easily digested, this is why.

The exact supplements you require depend upon your specific situation. It is recommended to consult an expert in medical care before you decide to take supplements in the long-term.

Additional Benefits

All over the globe, food companies have been required to include the nutritional content on their labels. In addition, many nations have their own standards of daily allowances for nutrition, that are intended to reflect the minimum amount of nutrients and vitamins that their population requires in order to avoid deficiencies as well as diseases.

Benefits of eating supplements that go beyond these levels are long debated. Some countries' suggested allowances and intakes are the upper and lower ranges of nutrition. These guidelines, at the lower side, represent an indication of the smallest amount required to avoid the development of deficiencies while on the other portion, it is the maximum amount that our bodies could manage before developing adverse negative effects from oversaturation of these minerals and vitamins.

The only thing we do not know are the proper quantities of these minerals and vitamins that our bodies require to operate in its optimal capacity. An investigation carried out in 2016 and later released in Nutrition and Metabolism revealed that metabolic and brain functions are able to be supplemented with micronutrients for adults, and even those who consider themselves to have a normal nutritional levels for the general population (Kennedy and co. (2016)).

The study results further noted that the taking of multivitamins/minerals is a low-risk way to both fill in any gaps in our nutritional coverage and as a possible benefit to improved mood, energy, and cognitive functions. Studies on the benefits are in line with these theories, however yet again, they confirm that supplements are not a substitute for the benefits of a healthy nutrition plan.

It's important to keep in mind the fact that all the studies conducted were done using healthy people in those who already have diverse, nutritious diets.

We should note that significant portions of the general population regularly take multivitamins/minerals and supplements not only to address nutritional gaps in their diet but to address stress, fatigue and improve their mental capacity. A study from 2010 that was published in Psychopharmacology specifically examined the effect on about 200 healthy males who were taking vitamins of the B complex that are vital for the process of metabolizing energy as well as vitamin C, as well as various minerals that enhance your immune system. Their results showed that participants in the group that were receiving multivitamins/mineral supplementation both performed better and rated themselves as feeling less mentally drained after completion of demanding cognitive tests. The study concluded that the healthy populace might benefit from higher levels of minerals and vitamins through direct diet-based supplementation. Particularly, the supplementation resulted in better ratings of stress levels physical health, mental health, energy levels, as well as improved performance through intense mental processing (Kennedy and co. (2010)).

Another study, that was conducted in 2010 one with about 200 healthy females, reached similar conclusion. Those in the group that was receiving multivitamins/minerals were less tired, and their moods less affected after performing extended tasks. As for their capability to work in a multi-tasking environment, they proved much more precise, and for certain activities, they performed faster and more precisely than others. Their results substantiated the notion that people who are healthy in the populace could gain from increased levels of vitamins and minerals through directly dietary supplements (Haskell and colleagues. (2010)).

This is just one reason why you should include nutritious foods that are rich in nutrients into your daily diet. A minimum of calories can keep you in good health However, it is important to achieve higher levels than the minimal. Our body and mind to be powerful engines.

Meal Planning

We first learned about the quantity factor, and then the quality, or nutritional aspect. Then, we must connect these two to create a dish. After all that what should we do to plan our meals?

Naturally, the final option is entirely yours However, I'll be sharing my strategies and take through a typical day in my life regarding my meals preparation to give you a good impression of how it all is a part of.

While some individuals like eating smaller meals during each day, I prefer to adhere to my 3 meals of the day including breakfast, lunch and dinner. There are a variety of reasons behind this. One is that I used to regularly and unhealthy snack throughout my day. I now attempt to avoid this sort of food routine. The second reason was that my brain was always stumbling across the room. It is my goal to make use of every opportunity to create a daily routine, as it helps me stay focused. In the end, I find it easier to do this. I prepare my own meals by having 3 set meals for the day makes it simpler to plan them and cook them.

My Meal Choice

When I wake up, I like to have a warm soups, as well as soft meals like yogurt which has been cooled to temperatures that are at room temperature. I like eating foods which are nutritiously balanced that are easy to digest, as well as lightweight enough to not get weighed down following meals. In the morning, I love to practice yoga or sit in meditation.

Personally, I've found it much easier to locate my place in the world by observing an unhurried daytime. For this reason I avoid things that are cold, hard or weighty. Naturally, this is my method. If you're like me, getting to a fresh, cold glass of water could provide the energy you require to start your daytime.

A few people would like to start each day with a hot cup of coffee. However rather than coffee I like a non-caffeinated hot drink that will keep me warm like hot lemon water or honey. If I'm under it, I love adding turmeric and ginger as antioxidants and astringent to hot water to make a soothing tea.

I've been a pscatarian, one who consumes all foods, but solely eats fish as a protein source, for approximately ten years. However, in recent times, if my body is feeling as though it requires a more powerful protein source, often after a workout that is intense and/or a long day, I'll eat an occasional serving of chicken. It's important to pay attention and be responsive to your body's requirements by listening to your body's needs.

My diet is heavily made up of vegetables, legumes as well as nuts. This is among reasons why I recommend using the Mediterranean food plan as a great start to learn how to cook healthy meals to eat, because it's like my current food habits as of now.

Sometimes, I use mushrooms in order to give a meaty taste to my meals. It gives me something to chew. The mushrooms are also nutrient-rich as they help with digestion as well as good health for the gut. Also, I enjoy enhancing my food using mild spice like cardamom cumin, coriander as well as cinnamon. There are times when I enjoy foods that are spicy and sweet, however personally, I feel them to be a bit too strong for my stomach which is why I like the mild spices.

In the evenings and lunches I generally eat whatever. I enjoy making myself meals, and I know enough about all the types of food and the nutrients I have to prepare the most balanced and healthy dinners. If I am feeling as though I'm in need of a more substantial food, I might start with a smaller starter. Most often, I'll have fresh cut avocados on a whole grain free, non-gluten (because due to my food intolerance) piece of lightly toasty bread.

The main ingredient of the meal is fresh vegetables that are often cooked along with a variety of nuts and served on top with brown rice. Brown rice that is whole grain is one of my favourite food items. Brown rice is, thankfully, gluten-free and I'm able to consume it without issue. If you're able to access the grains, I suggest cooking your rice using all-natural spices that give it an amazing aroma and a pleasant tasting. In accordance with what I'm craving at the time I like to pair it with cooked beans, mushrooms and a tiny portion of grilled fish fillet served on a side. These are side-meals that make good complements to the food, however they're only a small portion of a meal.

Portioning

Prior to learning how to manage my food intake properly, usually I'd eat until I was satisfied. This is how it works: you get hungry, consume food, and you are satisfied. Unfortunately, this is not the most effective approach to take even though it's the most convenient method. This approach is particularly poor when it comes to limiting your intake of calories since many calorific-rich sweet, fat-laden, and sugary meals aren't very filling.

The initial way to get rid of the eating habits was trying to divide my meals to ensure that they consumed me just half or sixty percent of my capacity. It also gives me the advantage of not making me feel full and uncomfortable afterwards and allowing me to go about my daily routine.

When I was able to prepare my own meals I began to cook my own food items. The process of weighing and recording my ingredients allowed me to keep track of precisely the amount of nutrients and calories I consumed. Over time, it got easy to assess the portion of my food items. I'm able take a look at the amount of fish on my dinner plate and remember its calories when I've prepared similar meals previously.

In recent days, I'm trying to incorporate more greens including spinach, lettuce and so on. in order to make my healthy meals. I also love sipping the water while eating. It is important to take my time eating, and I don't hurry through eating food. I prefer to slow down and take time to take my time eating and enjoying the meal. It makes me feel more full when I eat and keeps my from eating too much and snacking.

It's crucial to structure your lifestyle and diet to ensure that they can be sustained. Through changing my eating patterns and generally making my food more healthy, I've significantly enhanced my general well-being. I make sure to plan my meal and have a good picture of how many amount of calories I've consumed. I don't feel guilty if I'm tempted indulge in dessert or something sweet, because I keep track of those as well, even though it's rare that I indulge that.

Try New Things!

One last note: don't hesitate to explore different foods! I wasn't raised eating all the food I enjoy today. I had negative perceptions of a variety of seafood and vegetables due to one incident that I'm sure you're not alone. Don't let a negative memory hinder you from attempting them once more. There is an endless number of amazing recipes to suit various kinds of food. You can learn how to cook meals on your own and you'll be in a position to cook your meals according to the way you will love. Making your own food is the most effective and viable way to change your eating habits. A big part of this is the ability to continue increasing your menu of options. One method I use doing this is to shopping for seasonally-available fruits and vegetables. Vegetables and fruits are my main ingredients in meal, and I constantly test different recipes and methods of cooking the same, which makes it easier for me to not become bored with my food choices.

Chapter 13: Physical Exercise

As I started making adjustments to my lifestyle I started by changing the food I consumed and how I did it. I chose healthier choices I planned my meals and controlled my portion sizes. The advantages of a healthier eating plan were evidently fast.

In the early mornings I was a slog to rise. The process of waking up was a constant fight that cost me more than I did win. On days when I did manage to drag myself from beneath the blanket however, I felt tired. After I changed my eating habits, these issues began to diminish. I started waking up each morning feeling refreshed than I did the day before. The routine of waking up at the right time was becoming easy as I began to feel more alert and alert than I've ever experienced at the beginning of the day.

The effect grew throughout the course of time as I began enjoying some peace and quiet mornings. Beginning the day without stress and having fun throughout the day helped my mood significantly. I found it easier to concentrate on my task and didn't feel as if I was struggling to get up. Also, it easier to sleep in and the urge for an afternoon nap or to crash following a tiring day vanished. I was happier than I had for a while, and I felt more energetic to be motivated, as well as my spare time, which became motivations to keep my progress continuing.

Naturally, following the benefits I experienced with a balanced eating plan, the next stage for me was exercising. It was something I'd always vowed to do and yet, even though I was a lazy person sitting on the sofa but I never had an opportunity to begin. Perhaps it was anxiety about going to the gym only to be ashamed, or, most likely, I did not have the motivation or the motivation. After seeing the benefits of a few simple adjustments to my diet can have my life, I found myself possessed by an energy that was missing from me in the past. I was on the way to improve myself that could yield me immense fulfillment and joy. However, I'm advancing myself.

Prior to that, in Chapter 1 we looked at the importance of a balanced eating plan and how it directly influences your brain's power. It was my experience that eating a balanced diet is just one half of the equation. The other half is exercising. An appropriate diet coupled with regular workouts is crucial for maintaining and improving the health of your body. While our brains control every aspect of our lives that includes our thoughts to our actions as well as our bodies it is essential to be aware that they're in no way separate from one another. They function as collaborators. Our body's condition and health in general directly impact our brain health as well as our mental health.

Regular, consistent exercises that are routine and regular boost not only my physical fitness, but my mood as well. I went from being apprehensive about early morning run to wanting adrenaline. I had less stress and was generally more content. Diet and exercise made me manage my weight. My outlook about my circumstances improved since due to exercise and diet I was able to realize my own personal ways to effect changes in my own life, and realized that I was possessed of the power and potential to see through the cloud which had weighed my vision.

Why Is Exercise Necessary?

In full detail, the effect the diet we eat has on our lives. The physical health of us is similar. Health is maintained by an appropriate lifestyle and consistent exercise. As a lack of minerals or vitamins could cause significant problems to the cognitive function of our brain and our physical health, the lack of regular exercise will cause exactly the identical.

Dangers of Our Sedentary Lives

An active lifestyle is one which has little or no physical exercise. In the absence of exercise functioning of the body decreases. The muscles weaken even when they are not being used. One of the body's internal processes is to save energy. The heart also functions as a muscle. When the heart is weak it has a hard time pumping blood. Blood is the blood's vital sugar, which is the energy we require to perform. Additionally, there are other issues that may arise from an inactivity level including a myriad of health conditions that affect the heart and are chronic.

Today, it is all too simple and commonplace to slip into a lifestyle of sitting. The majority of modern day lifestyles are not much movement due to technology advances and evolving norms. When we work or at classes, we spend many hours at our desks. After we return at home, we sit on sofas or couches to unwind. When we travel between work, home or school, we're seated in busses, cars or train. If you are unable to find enough time to break your sedentary hours with exercising or sports then you'll begin seeing the signs of a lifestyle that is too sedentary for instance, the beginning of fatigue or a feeling of tiredness.

Lethargy

The signs of lethargy are fatigue, and also a feeling of a lack of motivation and an inability to do work. This can be indication of a diet that is not optimal which we've covered extensively in Chapter 1. The cause of fatigue can come from various other causes including sleeping insufficiently and, most often it is due to a lack of physical exercise or. The most common reason in our absence of physical movement is an external cause or tension.

If we're stressed and feel overwhelmed, we tend to retreat in our own space and search for ways for comfort. This can include lying down under blankets or on the sofa. Although this is a good way to reduce some of the symptoms, the more we remain in a relaxed condition, the more difficult it is to get out. The body is sucked into a state of apathy and don't have the energy to break from our comfortable zone. The key to breaking through that feeling of apathy is all about getting up and becoming engaged.

Physical Exercise

Exercise and being active is the next step in improving your brain power. It's not necessary to lift heavy weights or stress yourself out all day long however, incorporating at least 30 minutes of exercise every day could provide beneficial health effects.

There are a variety of forms of exercising, to the mind and body However, first I'd like to talk about the advantages of exercise and physical activity.

The Benefits of Getting Active

Exercise regularly, or any type of physical exercise is essential for preventing various chronic illnesses, particularly heart-related diseases. It can reduce your chance of suffering an accident that causes stroke. Exercises can also help strengthen your muscles, including your heart. This improves the quality of our lives and consequently directly affects the way we feel.

Exercise's benefits are not limited to the physical aspect of our well-being. Research has shown that consistent exercise can provide noticeable brain benefits starting from the age of 3 into old age, and could impact the overall health of our brains throughout our life (Macpherson and co. 2017, 2017).

Physical fitness is essential to the overall health of our bodies, as well as growing, development, and even aging. We'll look at some details about the impact exercise can have on our bodies to give us more understanding of how it affects the health of our body.

Muscles and the Heart

One of the most important methods that exercise directly affects health and fitness is by its interaction to our muscles. The muscles we have are vital to the daily routine of our lives. They allow us to move around and accomplish things. Have you ever thought about what we do to build muscles, and how they're capable of growing bigger?

Our muscles consist of numerous microfibers. If these fibers are damaged, such as when lifting heavy objects and the body repairs and replace damaged fibers with stronger and more powerful ones. This is the process that strengthens and builds our muscles however, it happens only when the fibers become damaged. If they're not injured, our body's muscles will remain the same as what it's currently got.

www.ingramcontent.com/pod-product-compliance
Lightning Source LLC
Chambersburg PA
CBHW071440080526
44587CB00014B/1923